A Guide to Transfer Factors and Immune System Health

2nd edition

Helping the body heal itself by strengthening cell-mediated immunity

Aaron White, PhD

A Guide to Transfer Factors and Immune System Health

2nd edition

Copyright © 2009 by Aaron White, PhD

ISBN: 1-4392-3262-8

ISBN-13: 978-1-4392-3262-0

First U.S. edition: September, 2007
Second U.S. edition: April, 2009
Updated December, 2009

BookSurge Publishing
North Charleston, South Carolina, U.S.A.

All books printed in U.S.A.

This book is dedicated with respect to Drs. Charles Kirkpatrick, Giancarlo Pizza, Paul Levine, Dimitri Viza, William Hennen and other medical doctors and researchers around the world who have devoted time to the study of transfer factors without need of fanfare or accolades from mainstream science. There can be little doubt that history will recognize the enormous importance of their efforts. Foremost, this book is for the late Dr. H. Sherwood Lawrence (1916-2004). It is regrettable he was not able to see this part of his work thoroughly vindicated and put to good use.

"In the realm of inductive science, the dominant paradigm can seldom be challenged in a frontal attack...and only what Kuhn calls 'scientific revolutions' can overthrow it...Because of the failure of medical science to manage the AIDS pandemic, transfer factor, which has been successfully used for treating or preventing viral infections, may today overcome a priori prejudice and rejection more swiftly."

- Dr. Dimitri Viza (1996)

Table of Contents

Chapter 5

Transfer factors were discovered in human blood cells but also are present in mammalian colostrum and in egg yolks. Recent advances in technology have made it possible to extract transfer factors from these sources and now they are available in supplement form. We will examine what makes them supplements rather than drugs. We will also explore practical issues regarding their use based on clinical reports.

Chapter 6

Transfer factors are useful adjuvants in the treatment of a wide range of viral, fungal and bacterial infections. They can be used to immunize the public against diseases. Based on existing research they represent a safe and effective means of boosting immune system health. We will explore the roles that transfer factors could play in disease management in the 21st century.

Appendix I

Appendix II

Introduction

> *"Transfer factors provide a 'databank' that helps our immune cells identify invading viruses and germs and then mount defenses against them."*
>
> - Dr. Kenneth Bock, MD and
> Dr. Steven Bock, MD (2007)

The 20th century was a golden era in modern medicine. Antibiotics emerged on the scene in the 1940s and dealt a serious blow to bacteria everywhere. In the late 1950s, two vaccines helped bring an end to the polio crisis and, by the late 1970s, a vaccination plan orchestrated by the World Health Organization succeeded in removing small pox from the world stage.

Though antibiotics and vaccines still play important roles in 21st century medicine, these and other approaches have begun to show their age. Chance mutations have allowed several disease causing bacteria to work around antibiotics. Drug resistant strains – such as those that cause tuberculosis, strep throat and gonorrhea – have been springing up with increasing frequency. Many bacteria, like *Borrelia burgdorferi* (Lyme), can shift into different forms, offering a unique means of evading detection and destruction.

In 2008, a highly anticipated HIV vaccine tested by Merck and the National Institutes of Health was found to increase the risk of contracting HIV. In early 2009, the Centers for Disease Control reported that the season's flu viruses were insensitive to the vaccine Tamiflu. Such failures came as health officials in both the U.S. and England pinned rising rates of measles infections on fear-driven declines in vaccination for measles, reflecting our continuing need for vaccines, or something like them, in the medical arsenal.

Since the mid-20th century, the pace of drug discovery has lagged far behind the pace of disease discovery. In recent years, due to public groundswell, several diseases in need of new treatments have demanded attention. Conditions like chronic Lyme, Babesia, Bartonella, PANDAS, ME/CFS, fibromyalgia, MS, recurring viral encephalitis and others. Such conditions are not helped by vaccines or short courses of antibiotics and are often treated with immunosuppressants, eventually causing further declines in health.

Many of our physicians still operate from antiquated perspectives on how diseases work – treating all bacterial infections with a few weeks of antibiotics and telling patients that anything viral will just run its course and go away. Patients with diseases involving multiple organ systems are routinely bounced from specialist to specialist, each treating only their part. Patients who do not improve after the first or second prescription are often dismissed as hypochondriacs or malingerers and referred to psychiatrists.

Any critique of American medicine must be tempered with several important asides. Medicine and the practice of medicine are not one and the same. American medicine, as a science, has long been on the cutting edge of disease discovery, characterization, treatment and prevention. Sadly, in the current climate, much of the science fails to influence the actual practice of medicine. Insurance companies and medical boards populated with eagerly compliant doctors drive practitioners to rely too strongly on pharmaceuticals – even for preventive care – and thus rob physicians of the opportunity to utilize more appropriate, often safer and more effective, treatment approaches in their practices.

By continually arming doctors with new medications and the findings of in-house science – not to mention trinkets, tickets and food – pharmaceutical companies create a false sense that they are providing MDs with everything they need in order to understand, diagnose and treat their patients' diseases. Beginning in 2009, an agreement signed by 40 drug companies will severely restrict the number of gifts and favors drug company representatives can give MDs. Hopefully this is the first step toward a period of renewed willingness to consider treatment options beyond the free-samples drawer.

Fortunately, several substances, natural and pharmaceutical, are in the pipeline as potentially powerful new weapons against disease and should provide physicians with a broader range of options in the near future. This book is about one emerging strategy with nearly 60 years of compelling science behind it – the use of immune messengers called transfer factors to treat and prevent viral and bacterial infections, boost overall immune system health and combat certain types of autoimmune conditions.

Transfer factors exist naturally in the body. They are made by white blood cells in the immune system and carry information about how to recognize cells infected with viruses (e.g., the herpes viruses, hepatitis C, HIV), mycobacteria (e.g., leprosy, tuberculosis) and cell-wall deficient forms of bacteria (e.g., Lyme). They are small strands of amino acids and bits of RNA that help white blood cells locate stubborn infections and heal them. Their presence after infections prevents re-infection. In other words, they play a direct role in creating immunity.

Transfer factors were discovered in the late 1940s when a young New York University immunologist named H. Sherwood Lawrence transferred immunity to tuberculosis from ill patients to healthy ones via extracts from the ill patients' white blood cells – findings confirmed repeatedly over the years. Because the molecule responsible for the seemingly miraculous effect was so difficult to identify, and the whole idea seemed so improbable at the time, Dr. Lawrence's early reports were not taken seriously.

Even without mainstream acceptance, research has come a long way in identifying the structure and function of Lawrence's transfer factors. Based on published literature and clinical reports it seems they offer a unique, powerful and safe means of immunizing the public against diseases and treating existing infections. Their discovery and mechanisms of action will be explored in Chapter 3.

It was nearly 20 years after Alexander Fleming's discovery of penicillin in the 1920s that technology finally allowed for mass production and the true arrival of antibiotics in the medical tool chest. (In the interim Fleming, like Ignaz Semmelweis who discovered the importance of hand washing before delivering babies, and Dr. Lawrence for his work on transfer factors, was chastised by the medical establishment.) For transfer factors, the mass production hurdle was crossed after it was discovered in the late 1980s that transfer factors are present not only in white blood cells, but also in mammalian colostrum and bird eggs, where they are normally passed from mothers to offspring. This process helps jumpstart newborn immune systems and educates them about disease-causing microbes encountered by the mother during her lifetime. In essence, genes code for an immune system capable of adapting to emerging threats. Transfer factors are a key part of that adaptive process. In Chapter 2, we will explore how immune information is transmitted through breast feeding and discuss whether the absence of important immune information in infant formula could explain why many of the health benefits of breast feeding are lost when synthetic milk is used instead.

Before the discovery of transfer factors in colostrum and egg yolks, transfer factors were extracted from human white blood cells and then injected into patients, making the approach expensive and impractical for routine use. Research conducted in the last few decades suggests that transfer factors generated by other mammals (e.g., cows) and birds (e.g., chickens) in response to pathogens are functionally, and perhaps molecularly, identical to those generated in the human body. Creative scientists took advantage of that fact and figured out how to extract transfer factors from cow colostrum and chicken eggs, both of which are considered foods under FDA guidelines. This bench work led to the sudden widespread availability of transfer factors in oral supplement forms during the late 1990s and is now creating a great opportunity to assess the value of transfer factor therapy for improving public health.

Recent research by the Russian Ministry of Health provides compelling reasons to believe that transfer factor therapy could have a positive impact on overall health and quality of life for patients with a variety of disorders. As summarized in a 2004 report on clinical studies of two commercially available transfer factor preparations,

> "TF and TF PLUS have marked immunocorrecting effects and are useful for their therapeutic and prophylactic effectiveness in various forms of infectious and somatic pathologies, which are accompanied by disease induced disturbances in immune status."

Chapter 4 contains an extensive review of studies and clinical reports in which transfer factors were used to treat and prevent a wide range of bacterial and viral infections. Because of their safety profile and apparent effectiveness, the risks of using transfer factors to fight diseases are small and the potential rewards great. The availability of transfer factors in supplement form, and their protection as supplements under law, will be the focus of Chapter 5.

Hundreds of studies have documented the safety and efficacy of transfer factors. They have been used to treat patients infected with ailments ranging from herpes to hepatitis and can protect those yet to be exposed to the agents that cause these conditions. The potential future of transfer factors in medicine will be examined in Chapter 6.

We will begin the book by taking a tour of the human immune system. Understanding disease states and making informed decisions about the use of supplements and drugs, as well as lifestyle changes, requires a basic understanding of how the immune system works. Next, we will explore the role that the immune system plays in keeping the body healthy and how taking care of the immune system can improve one's quality of life – physically, cognitively and emotionally. We will then turn our focus toward transfer factors and what research has to say about them.

It is the author's sincere hope that the material contained in these pages will peak your interest in the potential benefits of transfer factors for immune system health. If you are ill with an immune-related condition, hopefully the text will generate conversations between you and your family doctor or specialist about the possibility of adding transfer factors to your treatment protocol. If you are a doctor and are either currently unaware of transfer factors or simply want to learn more, the scientific reviews in Chapters 3 and 4 should be of help. In addition, Appendix I includes the titles and abstracts of 160 published papers on the subject spanning 60 years of research. Appendix II contains the New York Time's obituary for Dr. Lawrence, which captures the sheer scope of his contributions to immunology and medicine before his death in 2004.

Nothing in this book should be considered medical advice. The book is about the science behind one particular option for helping the body avoid or contend with illness. Like other health decisions, the decision to take products containing supplemental transfer factors should be made after careful consultation with, and under the close observation of, your physician. You just might have to catch them up to speed on the science first!

Chapter 1

Making sense of the immune system

The human body is made up of trillions of individual cells. Somehow, these cells manage to work together so that the enormous colony within each body functions as a single unified organism. Cells do this in part by forming tissues. Tissues then form organs. Sets of organs, known as organ systems, work together to accomplish common goals, like pumping blood around the body or digesting food and using it for energy.

There are ten organ systems within the human body, depending on how one categorizes things. These include the digestive, respiratory, circulatory, skeletal, muscular, endocrine, reproductive, excretory, nervous and immune systems. Each system has its own work to do, but all of the systems overlap and influence one another, as well. In the end, no disease state affects only one system.

It is the job of the immune system to protect the body from outside microbial threats, like bacteria, viruses, parasites and fungi, and to quickly get rid of body cells that become cancerous or are damaged in other ways. Doing so requires immune cells to be able to differentiate between *self* and *non-self* molecules and cells, and to get rid of non-self molecules and cells before they wreak havoc.

The immune system runs 24-hrs per day to keep the body safe. Unlike the digestive system and even the nervous system, the immune system never really gets a break. The warm and moist environment within the body provides a perfect breeding ground for bacteria and other organisms, meaning that the immune system must constantly be on guard. To understand how important the immune system is, one need only think of what happens to the body after death. When the immune system shuts down, the body is ravaged by microbes and decays.

The immune system is amazingly complex. Like the nervous system and the cardiovascular system, the immune system contains its own superhighway through which information flows. As blood is pumped throughout the body, the vessels become narrower and narrower until nutrients and fluid leak out through tiny porous vessels called capillaries. This clear fluid, called lymph, bathes the cells in the body, providing them with nutrients and oxygen, and carrying away waste products.

Eventually, lymph is either picked up by capillaries and transported back into the circulatory system or enters a vast network of tubules called lymph vessels. Lymph vessels carry the lymph to lymph nodes, where a wide variety of specialized cells screen the contents of the lymph looking for potential threats. In this way, lymph nodes are akin to checkpoints, where only friendly cells can pass. If foreign invaders or cancer cells are detected, an immune response is mounted.

The type of response initiated by the immune system and the various cells involved depends upon the nature of the threat. To understand this process, how different diseases happen and how the body fights them, let us look at some of the various cell types in the immune system, what they do, and how they do it.

1.1 Cells in the immune system

Lymphocytes

The immune system marshals an army of white blood cells with specialized functions. White blood cells are born in our bone marrow. We will discuss two major categories of white blood cells here. One of them, lymphocytes, consists of several variants, including *B-cells*, *T-cells* and *Natural Killer cells*.

Lymphocytes gather in various lymphoid organs, such as the lymph nodes mentioned above, the tonsils, the appendix (important for nurturing good bacteria in the gut) and the spleen (a specialized organ that filters blood looking for pathogens). Their activity is largely to blame for what people commonly call "swollen glands". While the name has no impact on how bad it hurts, the swelling actually occurs in lymph nodes, and there is really no such thing as a lymph gland.

Lymphocytes are always on the lookout for indications that the body is infected or that self cells have become cancerous or have died. Some lymphocytes, B-cells and T-cells, can distinguish between self and non-self cells based on the presence of *antigens*, characteristic molecules on the surface of pathogens or infected body cells. Others, like Natural Killer cells, spot intruders based on the *absence* of molecules normally expressed by healthy self cells.

Let us take a closer look at B-cells, T-cells and Natural Killer cells. Understanding them will help clarify the topic of immunity, which will be covered later in the chapter. It will also help us understand how some chronic disease states develop and what can be done to correct them.

B-cells

B-cells are lymphocytes that mature in the bone marrow itself ("B" for "bone marrow"). When a B-cell encounters an antigen, it generates an *antibody* for it. Antibodies belong to a family of proteins called immunoglobulins, often denoted by the letters "Ig". As the name implies, an antibody contains a region exactly the opposite of the antigen. This allows antibodies to attach to antigens. Antibodies can incapacitate the pathogens expressing the antigens and/or mark them for destruction by other immune cells.

Each B-cell can only produce antibodies that recognize one antigen. As such, the immune system has to produce thousands of different types of B-cells, each with the ability to produce antibodies for a specific threat. When an infection occurs, the appropriate B-cells begin cranking out antibodies in large numbers.

Sometimes, the antigens to which B-cells respond are not associated with a microbe but with dust, pollen, pet dander, or other allergens that evoke an immune response, causing the familiar symptoms of allergies.

B-cells are also responsible for cranking out *autoantibodies*, antibodies that stick to proteins on presumably healthy self cells and lead the body to attack itself, creating or contributing to autoimmune conditions. The real nature of autoantibodies, and autoimmune conditions, remains unclear.

T-cells

T-cells are lymphocytes that mature in the thymus, located behind the sternum ("T" for "thymus"). There are several types. We will discuss three types here – CD8+ Cytotoxic T-cells, CD4+ Helper T-cells and Suppressor T-cells.

Cytotoxic T-cells, also known as CD8+ T-cells, are like sharpshooters that accurately target infected cells. All viruses and some bacteria work by getting inside of healthy cells in the body. Once inside, they are out of the reach of antibodies. The only way to get rid of them is to kill the self cells in which they hide. Cells in the body are programmed to display antigens on their cell surfaces if infected. Cytotoxic T-cells are built to see those red flags and destroy the infected cells. How they kill infected cells is an interesting phenomenon and worth reviewing here.

There are two ways for cells to die – one is from direct injury of some kind and the other is from *apoptosis*, or programmed cell death. Apoptosis is very much like the self-destruct routines initiated toward the end of most science fiction movies. Apoptosis can occur naturally, as is the case when aging or unnecessary cells simply jettison their parts and disintegrate. It can also be triggered, and that is how Cytotoxic T-cells kill infected cells.

According to Charles Janeway from Yale and colleagues, Cytotoxic T-cells are highly efficient, and highly selective, killing machines. In their words (Janeway et al, 2001, first paragraph of section 8-24):

> "When cytotoxic T cells are offered a mixture
> of equal amounts of two target cells, one bear-
> ing specific antigen and the other not, they kill
> only the target cell bearing the specific antigen.
> The 'innocent bystander' cells and the cytotoxic
> T cells themselves are not killed."

While more tame, Helper T-cells, or CD4+ T-cells, play equally important roles in immune responses. These cells communicate with other immune cells to initiate and coordinate further attacks. Helper T-cells might stimulate antibody production by B-cells, alert Cytotoxic T-cells, or call in Natural Killer cells and phagocytes, which will be discussed shortly.

In essence, the activity of Helper T-cells represents a choice point for the immune system. As we will see, depending on how Helper T-cells react to an infection, the immune battle will head down one of two general pathways, called Th1 and Th2, the first involving the hunt for infected cells by Cytotoxic T-cells and the second involving the generation of antibodies by B-cells.

In addition to Cytotoxic and Helper T-cells, there is another type of T-cell called the Suppressor T-cell. Suppressor

T-cells, sometimes called Regulatory T-cells, or T*reg* cells, produce signals turning off the immune response. Such cells are important in calming the immune system down once the threat from a foreign invader has passed. Essentially, they serve as the brakes to an immune response. Suppressor T-cells play dual roles in autoimmune conditions. A healthy Suppressor T-cell response calms autoimmunity while weaknesses in Suppressor T-cells allow autoimmune conditions to worsen. Indeed, a weak Suppressor T-cell response could be the culprit in many conditions.

Natural Killer cells

Natural Killer cells represent another type of lymphocyte. Natural Killer cells are similar to Cytotoxic T-Cells in that they can identify threats and destroy them without calling for backup first. The key difference between Natural Killer cells and Cytotoxic T-cells rests in how they identify the threats. Cytotoxic T-cells look for antigens on the surface of cells. Natural Killer cells do not look for antigens. Instead, they look for cells that lack specific molecules that identify them as self cells. In other words, Cytotoxic T-cells look for evidence that a cell is officially *a non-self cell*, while Natural Killer cells look for evidence that a cell *is not a self cell*. A subtle, but extremely important difference that allows Natural Killer cells to destroy a very wide range of cells – essentially any cell that does not identify itself as a self cell – while Cytotoxic T-cells are only able to destroy cells with known antigens on their surfaces. In an Arnold Schwarzenegger movie, Cytotoxic T-cells would carry sniper rifles while Natural Killer cells would carry shotguns.

Natural Killer cells are called "Natural" Killer cells because they are ready to go to work killing bad guys as soon as they are born. They do not need to be educated and do not need to mature into a different type of cell before they can be effective.

Phagocytes

Phagocytes represent a second category of white blood cells involved in protecting the body from infections. These white blood cells are larger than lymphocytes and are capable of literally devouring potential threats. Phagocytes are antigen-presenting cells. That is, once they gobble up a foreign cell or object, they display the meal's antigens on their cell surfaces and then migrate into lymph nodes and present the antigens to lymphocytes (B-cells and T-cells), which then mount an attack.

While Helper T-cells are often credited with directing immune responses, it is important to note that phagocytes actually get things rolling. The signals they present determine what T-cells do next.

One type of phagocyte, the *macrophage* (a name that means "big eater"), plays a central role in the early immune response to a pathogen. Macrophages position themselves in areas of the body where microbes might enter, such as around the digestive tract, lungs and mucous membranes. Once an intruder is detected they gobble it up and sound the alert.

Some pathogens have stumbled across ways to use macrophages to their advantage. For instance, as we will discuss later in the book, HIV climbs inside of macrophages located in mucous membranes and hitches a ride to the lymph nodes where the virus then infects Helper T-cells and wreaks havoc on immune system health.

Macrophages are only able to alert T-cells about the presence of familiar pathogens with which the body has already dealt. On the other hand, phagocytes called *dendritic cells* are able to detect newly encountered microbes and then inform B-cells and T-cells about them. For this reason, dendritic cells are vital for the immune response to new infectious agents. As we will see, many infectious organisms work by hiding inside of healthy cells in the body. Chlamydia and Lyme, for instance. Dendritic cells are vital in the initial fight against these agents.

It was long thought that the brain did not contain immune cells. This was based mainly on the belief that the blood-brain-barrier adequately protects the brain and the rest of the central nervous system from invasion by pathogens, precluding the need for additional protection. We now know this assumption is wrong. Intruders do get into the brain, often very quickly, and the brain does contain immune cells – including a type of phagocyte called *microglia*. Like phagocytes in the rest of the body, microglia patrol the brain looking for foreign invaders or debris from dead and dying brain cells.

Granulocytes

Finally, the immune system contains several types of cells that fall under the category of granulocytes. Granulocytes are so named because they contain granules that can destroy microbes when they are injected into, or even sprayed onto, potential threats. One particular type of granulocyte, *mast cells*, plays a central role in the symptoms of seasonal allergies. We will return to a discussion of mast cells and allergies below.

1.2 Communication between immune cells

As we have seen, the immune system consists of a variety of cell types. In order for the immune system to initiate and coordinate attacks against pathogens, immune cells need to communicate with each other. They do this in part by presenting one another with direct evidence that an invasion is underway. For instance, when a phagocyte devours a threatening microbe, it displays antigens from the microbe on its cell surface and shows these antigens to lymphocytes. Lymphocytes then go to work labeling, tracking down and destroying the microbes.

Cells in the immune system also communicate with each other by producing and releasing a variety of proteins known as *cytokines*. The specific message that a cell conveys depends on the specific type of cytokines that it produces. For example, one subcategory of cytokines, called *chemokines*, are released from cells at the site of injuries, like a cut in the skin. Chemokines trigger inflammation and attract other immune cells to the area.

Another subcategory of cytokines, *interleukins*, can trigger the immune system to produce additional immune cells. They are called "interleukins" because of their ability to communicate messages between white blood cells (leukocytes).

As we will see later in the book, *transfer factors* represent a unique type of messenger used for cell-to-cell communication in the immune system. They are like a cross between interleukins and antibodies – carrying messages from cell-to-cell like interleukins and also binding to antigens like antibodies. These molecules, thought to be short strands of amino acids and bits of RNA, are created by Helper T-cells. They seem to facilitate the work of Helper and Cytotoxic T-cells by attaching to antigens on infected self cells and flagging the self cells for destruction. As such, they play important roles in helping the body deal with intracellular infections. More on transfer factors in a moment.

1.3 Common critters that threaten the body

Not long ago, just a few bacteria and viruses were recognized as threats to human health. On the virus side, chicken pox, measles, smallpox, polio, cold and flu come to mind. On the bacterial side, tuberculosis, leprosy, bacterial meningitis, staph infections and syphilis are all familiar conditions. It has become clear that the list of threats to human health is far longer than previously assumed. It has also become clear that infections probably account for many cases of cardiovascular disease, endocrine dysfunction, autoimmune conditions, neuropsychiatric conditions and more – disorders not previously believed to have an immune connection. The table on the following page contains an abbreviated list of agents now known to threaten health.

Some common pathogens

(Pathogen is from Greek *pathos*, suffering, and *gene*, to give birth to)

Type	Description	Associated diseases
Bacteria	Round, spherical or rod shaped single cell organisms without a nucleus. Broad category.	Staph, strep, gonorrhea, bacterial meningitis, salmonella, E. coli, bartonella, chlamydia
Virus	1000 times smaller than typical bacteria. Not living until inside a host cell. Contain genetic material and enzymes that allow them to take over the genetic machinery of host cells to make additional copies of themselves.	Flu, cold, human papilloma virus, measles, mumps, rubella, HIV, genital and oral herpes, viral meningitis, smallpox, Ebola, hepatitis C.
Mycobacteria	Type of bacteria that lives inside of host cells, including immune cells like macrophages.	Tuberculosis, leprosy, opportunistic infections in those with weak immune systems.
Mycoplasma	Type of bacteria that lacks a cell-wall making them difficult to treat with antibiotics. Live inside and outside host cells. When attached to outside of host cells they can trigger autoimmune conditions.	Pneumonia, pelvic inflammatory disease
Rickettsia	Type of bacteria often carried by ticks, fleas and lice. Grow inside of host cells. Can morph into several forms.	Rocky Mountain spotted fever, typhus, Oriental spotted fever
Spirochetes	Unique bacteria shaped like spirals. Flagella allow them to move in a spiral motion and penetrate hard to reach places in the body (joints, muscle, brain). Can shift into several forms - free spirochetes, cysts containing curled up spirochetes, granules containing information to create a large spirochete and cell-wall deficient forms that allow the spirochete to hide inside host-cells until ready to regenerate a cell membrane and move.	Lyme disease, syphilis, relapsing fever
Protozoa	Large parasitic organisms that cause a wide variety of diseases. Can exist inside and outside human cells. Often ingested in contaminated water or obtained from mosquitoes.	Malaria, toxoplasmosis, babesia, leishmaniasis, amoebic dysentery and giardia.
Nanobacteria	Tiny bacteria as small as some viruses. Sticky calcium coating leads to plaque formation. Calcium coating can be dissolved away with chelation therapy and the exposed bacteria are then sensitive to tetracycline.	Kidney stones, plaques in the cardiovascular system, bone spurs, anything commonly called a "calcium deposit"
Yeast	Fungus-like organism naturally present in the gut. Overgrowth leads the gut to become leaky allowing toxins to enter the body and evoke an inflammatory response. Overgrowth is triggered by antibiotics (which kill the healthy bacteria with which yeast compete), high sugar diet and/or immune weakness.	Systemic Candidiasis, vaginal yeast infections, thrush, intestinal yeast overgrowth.

Not included in the table is a specific category for cell wall deficient (CWD) bacteria. CWD bacteria, also called L-form bacteria, do not represent a specific type of pathogen, rather a particular state of existence common to many bacteria. Research on CWD bacteria dates back more than 100 years. Many bacteria have devised a survival strategy that involves shedding their easily detectable cell walls in order to hide inside, and alongside, healthy body cells until they are ready to rebuild their cell walls and emerge as fully formed organisms. This unique form of bacteria, regardless of the genus and species of the organism, poses unique threats to the body and unique hurdles to disease treatment and prevention. Indeed, the ability of some bacteria to retreat into the CWD form when threatened (as with antibiotics) could explain the relapsing and remitting nature of conditions like chronic Lyme, MS and other neurological conditions. As we will see, beating CWD forms of bacteria requires strong cell-mediated immunity. Transfer factors are immune messengers that help strengthen cell-mediated immunity and, research suggests, can help the body defeat CWD forms of bacteria.

The list on the previous page offers a glimpse into what the human immune system is up against in its fight to keep us disease free. Ultimately, strengthening the immune system is the best way to increase one's odds of avoiding or overcoming such infections. We humans did not make it this far with weak immune systems. Like the nervous system, the human immune system learns with experience and functions best when given proper nourishment and healthy environments that are not too clean or too dirty. Viruses and bacteria can be sneaky, but the immune system usually prevails when it is in peak form.

1.4 What does it mean to be immune?

The first time the body is exposed to a new virus or bacterium, an individual can become quite ill while the immune system struggles to react and get things under control. If healthy, the body will not be caught off guard twice. During the infection, the immune system learns to recognize the pathogen. The hope is that, if it comes back, the body will be able to contain it before a full-blown immune response is necessary. The process of fighting an infection and creating memories of the pathogen in order to fight more effectively the next time is called *immunity*.

The body has several means of protecting us from pathogens. The first line of defense is the outer shell – like skin, mucous membranes, nose hairs and fingernails. If pathogens get into the body, the next line of protection is what immunologists refer to as the *innate* immune system. This consists of dendritic cells, macrophages and other phagocytes, as well as Natural Killer cells. The innate immune system is considered unchanging. That is, experience does not change the basic function of these cells. Innate immune cells devour and kill foreign objects of all types. Some of these cells, the phagocytes, also present portions of the objects they eat to immature T-cells, called T_0 cells. This activates the next line of defense, known as the *adaptive* immune response.

Adaptive immunity is the process by which the body learns about and catalogues new foreign objects. This allows the body to track down an object floating around or hiding inside cells and deal with it quickly if it comes out of hiding or enters the body again.

Within the domain of adaptive immunity, there are two general strategies for dealing with infections, often categorized as humoral or *antibody-mediated* immunity and *cell-mediated* immunity. Antibody-mediated immunity is aimed at protecting the body from viruses and other specific pathogens found floating freely in blood and lymph. It occurs when B-cells learn about an antigen and create antibodies to it. A type of B-cell known as a memory cell is left behind after the battle and is able to quickly crank out antibodies if the host is ever exposed to the antigen again. The antibodies then cling to the antigen and disable it or flag it for destruction.

Cell-mediated immunity (a bit of a misnomer given that all immunity involves cells) is aimed at protecting the body from pathogens like viruses and bacteria that invade healthy cells. This type of immunity occurs when Cytotoxic T-cells learn to identify and directly destroy cells infected with pathogens. Both Helper and Cytotoxic T-cells with memory for the pathogen are left behind in order to launch an attack quickly the next time around. Evidence suggests that the number of memory cells left behind is proportionate to the number of cells involved in the initial immune response (Homann et al, 2001).

1.5 Th1 and Th2 immune response pathways

In the 1940s, immunologist H. Sherwood Lawrence discovered transfer factors, the topic of this book. He is best known for that innovation. His broader work on the roles of white blood cells in the immune system made an even bigger mark and contributed to speculation, in the 1980s, that adaptive immune responses can be divided into two broad streams – Th1 and Th2.

According to the basic model, Th1 immune responses lead to cell-mediated immunity, while Th2 responses lead to humoral or antibody-mediated immunity. The "Th" designation refers to the fact that Th1 (cell-mediated) responses are initiated by cytokines released from a subtype of T-cells called *T-Helper 1* cells, while Th2 (antibody-mediated) responses are initiated by cytokines released from a subtype called *T-Helper 2* cells.

The process appears to work as follows. A pathogen enters the body and eventually gets eaten by a phagocyte. The phagocyte presents antigens associated with the pathogen, along with specific cytokines, to a T_0 cell. The T_0 cell differentiates into a Th1 or Th2 cell, depending on whether the pathogen was found hiding inside a self cell (T_0 differentiates into Th1) or free-floating (T_0 differentiates into Th2). Next, the new Th1 or Th2 cell releases cytokines that trigger a domino effect leading to an immune battle and the symptoms of illness (such as inflammation, malaise, and so on). If successful, the response results in a resolution of the infection and immunity to the pathogen.

Cytokines released by Th1 cells – including IL-2, IL-12, interferon (IFN) γ, and tumor necrosis factor (TNF) α and β – play prominent roles in protecting the body from viruses and bacteria that get inside of healthy cells. Th1 cytokines trigger the recruitment of phagocytes and Natural Killer cells, which are efficient at finding and destroying sick self cells. Th1 cytokines also speed up the pace at which a phagocyte digests its meal. The impact of Th1 cytokines on phagocytes and Natural Killer cells highlights the interrelationship between the innate and acquired immune responses. Indeed, it appears that the Th1 response relies upon the activation of Natural Killer cells to be effective. While not technically part of the adaptive Th1 response, Natural Killer cells will be discussed as part of the Th1 response throughout the book. Cytokines released by Th1 cells also stimulate the actions of Cytotoxic T-cells, which hunt down and directly destroy cells infected with specific pathogens.

Cytokines released by Th2 cells – including interleukin (IL)-4, IL-5, IL-10, and IL-1 – promote the actions of B-cells, which in turn generate antibodies. Antibodies bind to free-floating pathogens, meaning those not hiding inside of cells. Antibodies and Th2 cytokines also stimulate activation of the complement system, a cascade of small proteins that help kill pathogens, enhance the ability of phagocytes to eat pathogens and remove immune complexes – the combination of an antibody and an antigen – from circulation.

Cytokines released by these two types of Helper T-cells work in mild opposition to one another. That is, cytokines released by Th1 cells can temporarily dampen Th2 responses and vice versa. For instance, if exposed to a pathogen that triggers a

Th1 response, the ability of the body to mount a Th2 response can be suppressed temporarily in order to route immune resources toward the Th1 battle. The opposite is also true. If all goes well, and the aggravating pathogen is defeated, the immune system returns to a balance of Th1 and Th2 activity. Unfortunately, some conditions involve chronic activation, or suppression, of one of these two categories of immune responses, wreaking havoc in the body and leaving the individual ill and susceptible to additional disease states.

In this book, we will focus primarily on what happens after Th1 cells are activated. The guiding hypothesis, one that could change as new research is published, is that the Th1 immune response leads to the generation of antibody-like peptides called *transfer factors*, which bind to antigens on the surface of infected body cells and help Cytotoxic T-cells identify their targets. Antibodies are at the core of the immune memories left behind after the Th2 response. It appears that transfer factors are at the core of the immune memories left behind after the Th1 response.

Some viruses and bacteria have evolved the ability to trigger an inappropriate immune response, thus forcing the body to over-produce cells incapable of destroying the pathogen and under-produce cells that are capable of destroying the pathogen. For instance, in order to fight HIV, a strong Th1 (cell-mediated) response is needed to detect infected cells and destroy them. However, the HIV virus is capable of triggering the release of Th2 (antibody-related) cytokines, thus suppressing the Th1 response, sending the body on a wild goose chase for antigens that can be targeted by antibodies, and thus avoiding destruction. Other viruses, such as HHV-6, one of the herpes viruses, can do something similar, as can the bacteria that cause Lyme disease. We will take a closer look at an example of how Lyme disease causes problems for the immune system in a moment.

It is important to recognize that the Th1/Th2 model of adaptive immunity is simplistic and that neither immune function nor diseases always obey the somewhat arbitrary Th1/Th2 dichotomy (Kidd, 2003; Steinman, 2007). The chemicals and cell-types involved in adaptive immunity are far too complex to sort into two categories. For instance, the model does not incorporate the recently characterized subtype of Helper T-cells, Th17 cells (Steinman, 2007). Nonetheless, the basic model is of great utility for trying to understand the process of disease and explore potential disease treatments.

To help the reader avoid confusion, it should be noted that some researchers use the designation Th1 to refer to *all innate immunity* and Th2 to refer to *all adaptive immunity*. In this outdated categorization of immune responses, Th1 responses are thought to trigger Th2 responses. In the present use of Th1 and Th2, both are subtypes of adaptive immunity and balance one another. This seems to be more in line with current data about how adaptive immunity actually works.

1.6 Vaccines and other issues regarding immunity

The speed and efficacy of an immune response against a pathogen is what differentiates those who *are* immune and do not get ill from those who *are not* immune and do get ill. The problem is that, in nature, immunity develops during an illness, and therefore can come at a great price. Vaccination is a process that allows humans to trick nature and develop immunity without becoming seriously ill (usually). It involves intentionally exposing the body to antigens or toxins expressed by a virus or bacterium in small amounts so that the immune system can learn about them, form memories for them, and deal with them quickly in the future.

In addition to dividing immunity into innate and adaptive and, more recently, dividing adaptive immunity into Th1 and Th2 responses, immunologists often refer to immune responses as *active* or *passive*. Both antibody-mediated and cell-mediated immunity are traditionally considered examples of active immunity because they usually develop as a result of experience. Passive immunity refers to immunity acquired from the mother during gestation or from the contents of colostrum after birth.

As we will see, transfer factors are capable of moving cell-mediated immunity from the active to the passive category. They literally *transfer* cell-mediated immunity from one person, or other animal, to another. As such, the recipient of transfer factors becomes immune to specific pathogens without having to mount their own initial immune response to it. This is one of several reasons why transfer factors have utility for public health and could usurp, or at least compliment, vaccines as the traditional source of intentionally induced adaptive immunity.

Immunity to viruses—Why do we become immune to some but not others?

Viruses are little clumps of protein containing some genetic material and the means to use that genetic material to hijack cells in our bodies. Once the body is infected with a virus, the immune system learns to identify antigens on the protein coat surrounding the genetic material (antibody-mediated immunity). It can also learn to identify antigens presented by body cells infected with the virus (cell-mediated immunity).

Some viruses do not change much from year to year. The virus that causes measles, for instance. As such, people tend to get measles only once before becoming immune to it. Unfortunately, many types of viruses, like those that cause cold and flu, are very shifty. They exhibit a high degree of *antigenic drift* — meaning that the surface molecules to which antibodies attach, and presumably the antigens displayed on the surface of infected body cells, change quickly. This makes it impossible to become completely immune to diseases like cold and flu, because the immune system has to learn to identify the antigens anew each time.

Is it possible to beat a relatively stable virus by immunizing enough people? Smallpox as an example

Until recently, the small pox virus was one of the most feared and deadly viruses around. It causes blistering over vast areas of the body and leads to a painful death. In 1796, Edward Jenner, a country doctor in England, performed the first ever vaccination to protect a human against a disease – in this case, small pox. Jenner noticed that people who milked cows were less likely to get small pox. He reasoned it was because these folks were being exposed to cowpox from the cows, and that the cowpox must be similar enough to small pox that the individuals' bodies were able to learn how to protect themselves against both diseases.

To test his hypothesis, Jenner rubbed puss from a cowpox sore into a scratch on the arm of an 8-year-old boy named James Phipps. A month and a half later he exposed James to the small pox virus to see if his strategy worked. It did! The boy did not contract small pox, ushering in a new option for preventing disease – vaccination. (The word "vaccine" actually comes from the Latin word for cow, "vacca.")

A unique strategy was used to get cow pox to America so that it could be used to inoculate colonists. Children were used to transport the virus. One would be infected before boarding ships headed for the New World. As that one began to heal, another child, and then another child, and so on, would be infected, until the voyage ended.

In the mid-20th century, Russia lobbied the World Health Organization (WHO) to make a push to eradicate smallpox by vaccinating portions of the population in each country where smallpox occurred. Nearly 20 years later, in 1977, the WHO announced that smallpox had become the first virus on earth to be eradicated by vaccinations. Only two known quantities of small pox remain on earth – one at the Centers for Disease Control in Atlanta, and one at the Moscow Research Institute for Viral Preparations. Let's hope they stay there!

The concept of *community immunity* and the continued relevance of vaccines

Several major infectious diseases were beaten into submission by vaccines in the 20th century. As the WHO worked to eradicate smallpox, similar efforts were underway to defeat the polio virus. The virus quickly enters the nervous system and damages brain cells involved in movement, including those that control breathing and walking. Polio incited panic in parents and children. In the 1950s and 60s, rivalry drove both Jonas Salk and Albert Sabin to develop effective polio vaccines, ending the disease's reign of terror in the U.S. and elsewhere. Among the lessons learned from these efforts was that vaccinating a certain percentage of the population can lead to protection for the whole clan, including those not vaccinated. Crossing the threshold leads to *herd*, or *community*, immunity. Different tipping points exist for different pathogens. For instance, to protect a population against mumps roughly 75% of the population must be vaccinated, while for polio the threshold for community immunity is closer to 85%.

The concept of community immunity has become quite relevant in recent years as concerns about mercury in vaccines and reports of side effects and links to developmental disorders have led many parents to opt-out of vaccinations for their kids. As a consequence, formerly quiescent diseases have re-emerged as public health scares. In 2008, England reported its highest number of new measles cases – 1,217 – in 13 years, pinning the spike on declining compliance with the recommended vaccine schedule. Indeed, health officials estimate that at least 25% of school-aged children in England are not fully vaccinated against measles, bringing the percentage dangerously close to the threshold for community immunity. A similar increase in measles infections occurred in the U.S. in recent years. In addition, the U.S. witnessed a minor resurgence of *Haemophilus influenzae* Type B (Hib) infections in early 2009. Hib is a bacterial infection that can be deadly in children. Rates plummeted 99% after introduction of a vaccine in 1990. The rise is associated with reduced vaccine compliance. Such reports can leave little doubt about the importance of vaccines, or something vaccine-like, in disease prevention.

As we will see, the discovery of transfer factors, and the development of techniques for generating pathogen specific transfer factors, should lead to vast improvements in our current approaches to immunizing the public against diseases.

Vaccines and the balance between Th1 and Th2 immunity

Vaccines play important roles in preventing the spread of infectious diseases. At present, we cannot do without them. However, the process by which they protect against diseases is out of step with the biology underlying the course of natural immunity and strains the balance between Th1 and Th2 immune responses in the body. As stated by retired Harvard biologist and renowned textbook author, John Kimball (2008):

> "Vaccines often elicit an immune response that does not actually protect against the disease. Most vaccines preferentially induce the formation of antibodies rather than cell-mediated immunity. This is fine for those diseases caused by toxins (diphtheria, tetanus), extracellular bacteria (pneumococci), even viruses that must pass through the blood to reach the tissues where they do their damage (polio, rabies). But viruses are intracellular parasites, out of the reach of antibodies while they reside within their target cells. They must be attacked by the cell-mediated branch of the immune system, such as by cytotoxic T lymphocytes (CTLs). Most vaccines do a poor job of eliciting cell-mediated immunity (CMI)."

The decision to utilize vaccines that preferentially activate antibody-mediated immunity was not made by choice but born of necessity. Indeed, early vaccine development occurred at a time when the distinction between Th1 and Th2 pathways was unknown. As discussed above, in the 1950s, vaccine researcher Jonas Salk helped bring an end to the spread of polio in America. He did so by exposing people to a deactivated form of the polio virus. His initial publicly tested version caused several hundred cases of polio and at least 10 deaths. This forced him to further deactivate the virus, which led to a safer vaccine. This was a miracle for public health – both physical and psychological. However, preventing the virus from causing intracellular infections meant that only the antibody-mediated wing of the immune system would be activated and the normal series of checks and balances between Th1 and Th2 immunity would be bypassed. The limitations, and implications, of the traditional vaccine approach are just now becoming clear.

Dr. Salk came out of retirement in the 1990s to tackle HIV via a therapeutic vaccine (Gorman and Park, 1995). The difficulties he encountered and the subsequent failure of his plan highlight the limits of vaccines for dealing with infectious agents like HIV. Clearly, vaccines cannot protect patients from every infectious disease. We will explore this issue further in Chapter 4.

1.7 Transfer factors

In subsequent chapters, we will discuss research on a fascinating type of immune messenger called transfer factors. As mentioned earlier, transfer factors appear to be short strands of amino acids and perhaps small bits of ribonucleic acid (RNA). It is thought that transfer factors are manufactured within Helper T-cells; cells that coordinate attacks launched by the immune system. Once released by Helper T-cells, transfer factors influence immune system activity in several ways. Their presence is read by other immune cells as an indication that a Th1-mediated immune battle is under way. This results in the birth of new Helper T-cells, Natural Killer cells and macrophages, the conversion of young lymphocytes into Th1-related immune cells, decreased levels of Th2-related cytokines, increased levels of Th1-related cytokines and a general strengthening of the Th1 response.

In addition, like antibodies, transfer factors bind to specific antigens. In the case of transfer factors, the antigens are located on the surface of infected body cells. Self cells infected with pathogens are programmed to display antigens from the pathogens on their cell membranes. New Helper T-cells use the presence of antigen-specific transfer factors to focus the immune response against particular threats. By sticking to antigens on infected cells, transfer factors effectively flag them for destruction by Cytotoxic T-cells.

In essence, transfer factors are the smaller siblings of antibodies, but operate to facilitate the destruction of infected body cells via cell-mediated immunity rather than the labeling of free-floating antigens via antibody-mediated immunity. Because transfer factors predominantly enhance Th1 immune responses, they hold tremendous promise in helping the body fight Th1 battles. This will be a topic of discussion throughout the book.

The B-cells that make antibodies contain receptors for antigens on their cell membranes. Antibodies are free-floating versions of the receptors present on the B-cells that make them. T-cells also contain receptors that bind to antigens. It is possible that transfer factors are free-floating versions of the receptors present on the T-cells that make them (Kirkpatrick and Rozzo, 1995). This is one of several questions awaiting further research.

During the natural course of an infection, transfer factors aimed at specific viruses and bacteria are created. As reviewed in Chapter 3, when taken from an ill patient and given to a healthy person, pathogen specific transfer factors literally *transfer* cell-mediated immunity from the ill patient to the healthy person.

The recipient's body simply responds to the transfer factors as though they were created internally.

Research reveals that transfer factors from cows and chickens are similar, perhaps identical, to those generated in the human body, making it feasible to generate pathogen specific transfer factors for human consumption using cows and chickens – a development with tremendous potential to improve public health and prevent the spread of disease.

In summary, transfer factors are made by white blood cells during the course of fighting intracellular infections. They draw resources to such battles and trigger changes that strengthen the Th1 immune response in general. Given in supplement form, they can be used to help the body beat infections. Given before infections occur, they act in a manner similar to vaccines and protect the body from becoming infected. While antibodies are at the heart of antibody-mediated (Th2) immunity, transfer factors hold the key to cell-mediated (Th1) immunity.

1.8 When things go wrong

Allergies

The process that leads to the annoying symptoms of allergies reveals a great deal about how the immune response works, and how it can cause nagging problems when it is triggered inappropriately.

When one is first exposed to a potential allergen, such as pollen, ragweed, or mold, B-cells create a particular type of antibody, known as IgE (immunoglobulin E) for the substance. Some of these antibodies attach to mast cells, a specific type of granulocyte that is concentrated in the lungs, nose, mouth, skin and gastrointestinal tract. When the body is exposed to the allergen, such as by inhaling it, it binds to the complementary antibodies and triggers the mast cells to release histamine contained in granules inside the cells. Histamine causes the inflammation and related symptoms associated with allergies. Indeed, one common strategy for alleviating allergies is to take "antihistamines" to block the effects of the histamine signals.

Allergens are not always inhaled, but are sometimes swallowed or simply absorbed through the skin. Normally, large molecules from food are broken down during the process of digestion prior to being absorbed into the body. In people with a condition known as *leaky gut*, such molecules get into the body without being broken down. This appears to be the process that leads to peanut allergies, and other food allergies, in some children. Presumably, proteins from peanuts are absorbed into the body where they trigger an immune response leading to antibody production and an allergic reaction upon subsequent exposure.

Autoimmune conditions

As we have discussed, one of the main tasks of cells in the immune system is to distinguish self from non-self cells. The long-held view of autoimmune conditions posits that, when mistakes are made, and self cells are mistaken for non-self cells, B-cells generate antibodies, called *autoantibodies*, that lead the body to attack itself. Conditions considered to result from autoimmunity include MS, lupus, Hashimoto's thyroiditis, Type I diabetes, and others.

In many cases, it is possible that what appear to be autoimmune responses are actually immune responses aimed at currently unidentified intracellular pathogens, such as forms of mycobacteria, CWD bacteria or even nanobacteria (bacteria-like life forms smaller than some viruses). For instance, in a paper entitled, "Sarcoidosis succumbs to antibiotics – Implications for autoimmune disease," Marshall and Marshall (2004) discuss evidence that the autoimmune condition, sarcoidosis, might actually be caused by CWD bacteria. If so, perhaps other autoimmune conditions are also caused by infections.

Support for the position of Marshall and Marshall comes from the fact that some autoimmune conditions are characterized by an abundance of Th1 cytokines, particularly interferon gamma (INFγ), which recruits phagocytes and Natural Killer cells to the site of an infection. It is possible that the Th1 response triggers an ongoing battle in which infected self cells are destroyed. What are commonly referred to as autoantibodies could be antibodies generated against fragments of the dead self cells resulting from the Th1 immune battle.

Some researchers speculate that pleomorphic bacteria, such at *Borrelia burgdorferi*, which causes Lyme, attempt to evade detection by coating themselves in the membranes of host cells. Theoretically, this could lead the body to make antibodies against the pathogen that ultimately lead the body to attack the membranes of self cells.

A pathogenic basis for autoimmune conditions could explain their diverse presentations and the fact that autoimmune conditions have been linked to Th1 hyperactivity, Th2 hyperactivity and simultaneous Th1/Th2 hyperactivity. The nature of the immune imbalance could vary based on the type of infection.

It is also possible that, ultimately, autoimmune conditions are not rooted in Th1/Th2 imbalances at all. Indeed, recent studies suggest that Suppressor T-cells, discussed earlier, might hold the key to calming autoimmune conditions. These cells serve as the brakes to immune responses. What appear to be Th1/Th2 imbalances could be secondary to weaknesses in Suppressor T-cell activity (Leceta et al, 2007). Further, the recently characterized subtype of Helper T-cells, Th17, could play important roles in autoimmunity, as well (Steinman, 2007).

Research suggests that one variant of transfer factor activates Suppressor T-cells and could be useful for some autoimmune conditions. Other treatments that activate Suppressor T-cells, such as vasoactive intestinal peptide, also could be helpful (Delgado et al., 2005). More on autoimmune conditions in Chapters 3 and 4.

Immunodeficiencies

When the immune system is missing one or several components, the body is left poorly protected and a variety of disease states can result. Some of these conditions are acquired, while others are inherited. The most notable of the acquired immune conditions is Acquired Immune Deficiency Syndrome (AIDS). AIDS results when the HIV virus infects T-cells and uses them as breeding grounds for viral replication. It does so by inserting new genes into the DNA of the T-cells, turning the T-cells into HIV factories. The virus also triggers the release of cytokines that trick the body into thinking it should mount a strong Th2 (antibody-mediated) immune response when a strong Th1 (cell-mediated) response is needed. Thus, the virus simultaneously replicates and disables a critical component of the immune response, leaving the host susceptible to a wide range of additional disease states, including cancers (e.g., Kaposi's sarcoma) and bacterial infections (e.g., pneumonia). People who die from AIDS do not die from the HIV virus itself, but from secondary infections that result from the actions of the HIV virus.

When the immune system gets stuck in the "on" position

Several disease states involve an inability of the immune system to effectively deal with disease causing pathogens, leading to chronic immune activation and the complications that result while simultaneously leaving the host vulnerable to other infections. As discussed previously, this appears to be the case in some, perhaps all, autoimmune conditions. The individual might not be missing immune system components, but the components that the person has are insufficient or out of balance. Such appears to be the case with Myalgic Encephalomyelitis /Chronic Fatigue Syndrome (ME/CFS), a condition known by several other names, including Chronic Fatigue Immune Dysfunction Syndrome (CFIDS) and Chronic Fatigue Syndrome (CFS).

Many individuals with ME/CFS test positive for active infections with a variety of viruses, including HHV-6, one of the eight known herpes viruses. The immune system appears to get stuck in the on position in an effort to eradicate the viruses. This could stem from an insufficient Th1 response at a time when that is just what is needed. Because the immune system cannot overcome the pathogens, the person feels chronically ill. As the immune system attempts to deal with current infections, the host is left vulnerable to additional infections and the chronic, but insufficient, immune activation is simply perpetuated.

The initial trigger for this vicious cycle is unknown and likely varies from person to person. Logically, it could stem from innate weaknesses in the Th1 (cell-mediated) immune response. As such, the viruses might not cause the initial problems. Rather, their presence is an indication of the underlying problems.

It is also possible that the cycle begins after a major immune battle with a virus or bacterium. In the wake of the battle, while the immune system is recovering, a window of opportunity might exist for additional infections to occur and for the immune system simply to become swamped.

Regardless, chronic immune activation, and chronic immune suppression, seem to occur at the same time in some ME/CFS patients, resulting in an ineffective immune response that leaves the person feeling ill day after day.

Intestinal dysbiosis – Can't we all just get along?

The intestines represent 25+ feet of mucous, acid and bacteria covered fleshy tubing that can be classified as existing inside or outside the body depending on the open or closed states of a few sphincters. Ingested substances are blended together with acids and enzymes in the stomach before being emptied into the small intestine, measuring roughly 20 feet long and 1.5 inches wide. Here and in the large intestine, measuring somewhere around 5 feet long and 3 inches wide, food molecules are torn apart, modified and absorbed into the body. A branch of the nervous system, the enteric nervous system, one separate from but influenced by the sympathetic and parasympathetic branches of the peripheral nervous system, causes muscles around the intestines to undulate ensuring that food processing continues to move in the right direction.

The intestines have nearly as much surface area as the entire human body. Far more bacteria and other micro-organisms exist in the intestines than there are self cells in the whole human host. Cells in the intestinal microbiome (all cells, host and non-host, in the intestines) play critical roles in the absorption of fats and carbohydrates, promote the growth of body cells lining the intestines and even create some vitamins, like thiamin (B1). More than 500 species of bacteria and other organisms are thought to co-exist in an "I'll scratch your cell membrane you scratch mine" kind of relationship with cells that represent the human side of the equation. When this symbiotic relationship goes awry, the health of all living things in the bacterial colony and the human host can be put at risk.

Hundreds of species of bacteria compete with a few species of yeast for resources in the expansive, warm moist world of the intestines. Normally, the bacteria dominate, in part by releasing their own antimicrobial peptides, and help keep the potentially pathogenic yeast at bay. There are several scenarios in which the yeast can begin to gain some ground, take over territory in the intestine, and wreak havoc for the human host. In one scenario, antibiotics taken for bacterial infections inside the human host kill off large swaths of bacteria in the intestines, creating a window of opportunity for the yeast to seize territory. In another scenario, yeast simply thrive on diets full of sugar and get a foothold. Once established, colonies of yeast grow roots called *rhizomes* that can puncture the walls of the intestines and allow other molecules, and perhaps entire organisms, to gain entry into the body itself. Food allergies are one potential consequence. There are others.

During infancy, gut microorganisms are given a free pass by the immune system. As long as they stay in the gut, the immune system leaves them alone. However, once they, or even portions of them, enter the body a full-blown immune response can result. Of particular concern is the likelihood that the leaky gut caused by yeast overgrowth allows lipopolysaccharides (LPS), a major membrane component of bacteria in the gut and elsewhere, to enter into the body. Once in the body, LPS acts as a potent toxic agent, triggering a widespread inflammatory immune response. Sick behaviors (e.g., withdrawal, fatigue) and the accompanying emotions (e.g., anxiety, depression) would be expected to follow. While treatments aimed at the symptoms could prove useful in the short-term, only destroying the yeast and repopulating the gut with symbiotic bacteria can resolve the problem. Fortunately, intestinal yeast levels are measured in several laboratories and antifungals and probiotics can be used to destroy the yeast and repopulate healthy bacteria.

Immune dysfunction caused by evasive bacteria – Lyme disease as an example

In the 1980s, as the HIV/AIDS epidemic took center stage, a poorly understood tick-borne infection was causing concern, particularly in the northeast. Ground zero, at least with regard to diagnoses, was Lyme, Connecticut. Lyme disease, as it is now known, is caused when the bacterium, *Borrelia burgdorferi* (Bb), or one of its close relatives, makes its way into human hosts, typically via deer ticks.

Lyme is caused by a spirochete – a corkscrew shaped organism that can shift into various forms at will (see Rubel, 2003, in the references for a fantastic overview of Lyme and its various forms). In the spiral form, the organism is propelled by flagella and can burrow deep into

> *I have found these granules* [from spirochetes] *to be resistant forms and their presence in countless numbers in the tissues might explain part of the mechanism of relapse and the difficulty of curing completely some of the more chronic spirochaetal infections, as, for example, syphilis and yaws.*
>
> - Balfour, 1911

muscle tissue, the fluid in joints, the central nervous system, and virtually anywhere in the body it chooses to infiltrate. This form is susceptible to antibiotics. However, several other variants of the organism are difficult to beat with antibiotics and can go undetected by the body's own defenses.

It is common for the spirochete to form buds, or granules, that contain sufficient genetic information for the buds to re-form into individual spirochetes. Full grown spirochetes are also known to wind themselves into tight balls and form cysts. These cysts can exist both outside and inside of host cells, are difficult to detect and insensitive to most antibiotics. While inside the cysts, the bacteria multiply in such a way that the new spirochetes can have different antigens in their cell membranes than the previous wave of adult spirochetes, making it even harder for the body to detect the infection. Lyme spirochetes, like many other organisms, are also known to form colonies covered by a slime-like coating called extracellular polymeric substance (EPS), which can prevent antibiotics from reaching bacteria at the core. Finally, it appears that spirochetes can hide inside of cells by shedding their membranes and existing in a cell wall deficient (CWD) form, also called an L-form.

Interactions between the impressive array of bacterial forms Bb takes and the immune system help explain the various symptoms seen in Lyme patients. Rosner (2007) suggests the spirochete form of Bb could be responsible for the flu-like symptoms many patients experience while the cystic form and CWD form could mimic conditions ranging from MS to ME/CFS. As can be seen in the general symptom checklist on Page 41, the symptoms of Lyme are incredibly diverse and likely depend on both the locations of the infection and the form the bacteria take in those different areas. Infections in brain areas involved in emotions will have different effects than infections in brain areas involved in movement, and both will manifest in symptoms far different from infections in the heart, prostate or joints.

Some patients test positive for Bb but are asymptomatic. Some develop illness and are able to beat Bb infections early with the help of antibiotics. For others, a few weeks of antibiotics could kill a large enough number of adult spirochetes to ameliorate acute symptoms and lead to the mistaken conclusion that the patient is cured. For them, the granules, cysts and CWD forms of the bacteria that remain eventually lead to a resurgence of free spirochetes and a return of symptoms. Indeed, some antibiotics likely spur spirochetes to retreat into protective forms until conditions are more favorable. As such, Lyme disease often defies the simple "get bacteria take antibiotics for a few weeks" mentality of modern medicine.

A clue to what is needed to defeat Bb comes from the ways in which Bb attempts to influence the immune systems of infected hosts. The bacterium favors a Th2, or antibody-mediated, immune response and, at the same time, has developed mechanisms for preventing easy detection by antibodies. Like HIV, Bb suppresses the ability of host cells to release cytokines that evoke cell-mediated activity. The one-two punch on Th1 and Th2 immunity allows Bb to hide in plain sight. In addition, when the level or "load" of bacteria is high, Bb directly attacks and damages the immune system, making it even harder to detect and eradicate. According to the International Lyme and Associated Diseases Society (ILADS) (Burrascano, 2002):

> "Studies have shown that higher loads [of Bb]...begin to clinically impact the immune system, with invasion and killing of B- and T-lymphocytes, including Natural Killer cells, and inhibition of lymphocyte transformation and mitogenesis... There is evidence that B. burgdorferi [Bb] can remain viable within cells, such as macrophages, lymphocytes, endothelial cells, neurons, and fibroblasts...In addition, Bb can coat itself with host cell membranes, and it secretes a

glycoprotein that can encapsulate the organism... In theory at least, these coatings interfere with immune recognition, thus affecting the clearing of Bb, and also cause seronegativity."

Once the immune system suffers insults like the loss of critical lymphocytes and inhibition of the conversion of new white blood cells into active immune cells, it is difficult to imagine how the body could ever get the upper hand. By tricking the immune system and diverting its attention away from detecting and destroying infected cells, the bacteria and other pathogens conveyed by the tick bite avoid being wiped out. The patient can remain persistently or intermittently ill even when blood tests fail to detect evidence of an active infection.

Reports suggest that, within 12 hours of infection, the Bb spirochete can enter the central nervous system (the brain and spinal cord), making it even more difficult for the body, no matter how healthy it is, to launch an effective attack. Indeed, the cyst form of Bb has been found hiding in a brain structure known as the hippocampus (Mac-Donald, 2007), which plays a prominent role in creating memories for facts and events (Best and White, 1998). The presence of Bb in the hippocampus could help explain the memory problems suffered by many Lyme patients. MacDonald (2007)

> *These most recent findings do confirm the development of membrane-derived cysts, blebs, spherules, vesicles and the potential transformation to motile, helical spirochetes, not as part of a complex developmental cycle... but rather as a 'survival mechanism' of spirochetes to overcome or escape unfavorable conditions... It is tempting to speculate... that the survival mechanism of spirochetes is responsible for the diverse pathology of these organisms as well as for their ability to survive as cystic forms thereby producing prolonged, chronic and periodically recurrent disease.*
>
> - Burgdorfer, 1999

suggests that Bb in the hippocampus could contribute to the progression of Alzheimer's disease.

It is well known that syphilis, also caused by spirochete bacteria, can trigger debilitating problems with thought and mood and can lead to full-blown mental psychosis in later stages. It should not be surprising that untreated or poorly treated infections with Bb can cause similar problems. Again, according to ILADS (Burrascano, 2002):

> "It is clear that in the great majority of patients, chronic Lyme is a disease affecting predominantly the nervous system."

At present, current medical dogma holds that chronic Lyme does not exist. Short-courses of antibiotics are presumed to kill all of the bacteria and any leftover symptoms are attributed to some sort of "hit and run" effect of the infection. Such views persist despite more than a century of evidence that spirochetes have mastered the art of evading detection and destruction. Fortunately, such dogma is slowly giving way to reason and the recognition of chronic Lyme as a persistent infection. Indeed, in May of 2008, the national doctor's group, *Infectious Diseases Society of America*, was forced to revisit its position that chronic Lyme does not exist following pressure from Connecticut's attorney general.

The impact of stubborn medical dogma on Lyme disease treatment, and the refusal of highly educated researchers and medical doctors to recognize that Lyme, like syphilis before it, can be difficult to eradicate from the body, is captured in a letter written by Marjorie Tietjen – patient, advocate and journalist – and posted on the website of the Canadian Lyme Disease Foundation:

> "One of the main forces behind the non-treatment of Lyme is Yale's stance that 3 to 4

weeks of antibiotic treatment is almost always sufficient to produce a cure. Certain doctors at Yale contend that after the 30-day treatment period, if one still has the exact same symptoms, it is no longer active chronic Lyme but is now suddenly an autoimmune disorder. They have no proof to back this up and this was made evident when they did testify at our first Lyme hearing several years back. Perhaps this is why they were reluctant to attend our most recent hearing. Many patients who go to Yale for help with suspected Lyme are being diagnosed with Multiple Sclerosis, Fibromyalgia, Chronic Fatigue syndrome, ALS and even Lupus. Yale evidently feels there is no such thing as chronic active Lyme Disease."

Assuming one can find a doctor to treat chronic Lyme, the typical treatment approach involves a long-term (six or more month) course of antibiotics, sometimes intravenously, along with drugs specifically targeting the cyst form of the bacteria. An antifungal is often recommended to prevent yeast overgrowth caused by the death of healthy bacteria in the gut during antibiotic therapy. There are several non-traditional treatment protocols available involving everything from increasing oxygen levels in the body to taking various herbal antimicrobials. Regardless of how one treats Lyme, of particular import is identifying and working to correct the damage done to various organ systems during the course of the Bb infection so that the body can heal and regain the upper hand. This often includes correcting hormone imbalances and addressing psychiatric symptoms.

Lyme patients are well aware that this can be a difficult infection to beat and that it requires a doctor who understands the disease. Such doctors are known to patients as Lyme

Literate MDs, or LLMDs. (See www.ilads.org for more about treating Lyme and to locate LLMDs.)

Lyme Disease symptom checklist from ILADS (www.ilads.org)	
1. Unexplained fevers, sweats, chills, or flushing	23. Neck creaks and cracks, neck stiffness, neck pain
2. Unexplained weight change (loss or gain — circle one)	24. Tingling, numbness, burning or stabbing sensations, shooting pains, skin hypersensitivity
3. Fatigue, tiredness, poor stamina	25. Facial paralysis (Bell's Palsy)
4. Unexplained hair loss	26. Eyes/Vision: double, blurry, increased floaters, light sensitivity
5. Swollen glands: list areas	27. Ears/Hearing: buzzing, ringing, ear pain, sound sensitivity
6. Sore throat	28. Increased motion sickness, vertigo, poor balance
7. Testicular pain/pelvic pain	29. Lightheadedness, wooziness, unavoidable need to sit or lie down
8. Unexplained menstrual irregularity	30. Tremor
9. Unexplained milk production; breast pain	31. Confusion, difficulty in thinking
10. Irritable bladder or bladder dysfunction	32. Difficulty with concentration, reading
11. Sexual dysfunction or loss of libido	33. Forgetfulness, poor short term memory, poor attention, problem absorbing new information
12. Upset stomach or abdominal pain	34. Disorientation: getting lost, going to wrong places
13. Change in bowel function (constipation, diarrhea)	35. Difficulty with speech or writing; word or name block
14. Chest pain or rib soreness	36. Mood swings, irritability, depression
15. Shortness of breath, cough	37. Disturbed sleep — too much, too little, fractionated, early awakening
16. Heart palpitations, pulse skips, heart block	38. Exaggerated symptoms or worse hangover from alcohol
17. Any history of a heart murmur or valve prolapse?	
18. Joint pain or swelling: list joints	
19. Stiffness of the joints or back	
20. Muscle pain or cramps	
21. Twitching of the face or other muscles	
22. Headaches	

Ultimately, only the human body itself can defeat Bb, though antibiotics and other medications certainly help tilt the odds in the body's favor. Many Lyme sufferers go long periods between bouts of symptom flare-up, though others suffer debilitating symptoms year round. The difference could rest in the ability of the host immune system to corral the bacteria and force it to stay in hiding, quickly pouncing on any spirochetes that emerge from granules, cysts or slime covered colonies. It is comforting to think that the body gets rid of all traces of the viruses and bacteria that infect us and in some cases it does. With pathogens like Bb, the herpes viruses, malaria and tuberculosis, an effective immune system beats the agents into submission and keeps them there – hopefully forever – so that they can do no harm. Without an effective immune system, active infections can become persistent or recurrent.

Based on how transfer factors affect immune system health, they could serve as powerful allies in the treatment of Lyme. In a paper published in the prestigious *Proceedings of the National Academy of Sciences*, Tupin et al. (2008) report that Natural Killer cells, key components of the Th1 response, play a primary role in preventing joint inflammation during the course of Lyme infections in mice. The authors conclude that the outcomes,

> "…counter the long-standing notion that humoral rather than cellular immunity is sufficient to facilitate Lyme disease resolution."

Transfer factors trigger increases in Natural Killer cell levels and augment the killing efficacy of Natural Killer cells that already exist. They boost levels of Th1 Helper T-cells, macrophages and dendritic cells and should pull the body away from the Th2 (antibody-mediated) dominant state evoked by the Lyme bacteria, if such a state occurs. Broad-spectrum transfer factors boost immune system health in general and could be quite beneficial in the treatment of Bb and other stealthy infections. In cases where the Th1 response is stuck in the on position as it attempts to fight the various forms of Bb, transfer factors could help push the battle over the top by strengthening the response. The changes initiated by transfer factors would help prepare the body to deal with spirochetes as they re-emerge from the cyst form, which is one of the underlying culprits in the chronic nature of the disease, and to deal with adult spirochetes that develop from granules.

Targeted transfer factors – those generated against the various incarnations of the Lyme bacteria – could be particularly beneficial for helping the body locate and destroy the intracellular CWD form of Bb as well as spirochetes that burrow into hard to reach places like joints and the brain. It seems that Lyme is a disease best met with a strong cell-mediated immune response. Transfer factors should override efforts on the part of Bb to thwart such an immune response and help the immune system overcome the illness in the event that the Th1 response is elevated but insufficient in later stages of the infection. The combination of antibiotics and transfer factors could be particularly effective against Bb and other bacteria capable of morphing into different forms and lying dormant.

Research on the utility of transfer factors in disease treatment and prevention will be the focus of Chapter 4. At present, there are no published studies assessing the effectiveness of transfer factors against Lyme disease, though logic supports their use and personal reports from physicians and patients who have tried them are quite promising. In his 2008 report, "Advanced topics in Lyme disease: Diagnostic hints and treatment guidelines for Lyme and other tick borne illnesses," Lyme treatment pioneer Joseph Burrascano MD writes, "Personal experience made me a believer in transfer factor therapy. For Lyme patients...I have found them to be surprisingly effective in making the very ill respond better to treatment."

1.9 Summary

In this chapter, we took a tour of the immune system and how it works. Here is a summary of what we covered:

- The immune system consists of a wide variety of cells and organs that monitor the contents of the body to identify and destroy potential threats.

- Immune cells are born in bone marrow and mature into various cell types. T-cells mature in the thymus while B-cells mature in the bone marrow itself. Both are lymphocytes.

- B-cells produce antibodies that attach to molecules, called antigens, on the surface of free-floating microbes and either disable them or mark them for destruction. They also play roles in allergies and autoimmune conditions.

- Phagocytes, including macrophages and dendritic cells, are large white blood cells that gobble up microbes and infected cells and present their antigens to lymphocytes so that they can coordinate an immune response.

- Helper T-cells recognize foreign threats via antigen receptors on their cell membranes and then organize the appropriate immune response to take care of the threats

- Cytotoxic T-cells look for antigens on the surface of infected body cells and then directly destroy the cells.

- Suppressor T-cells turn off the immune response once a battle is complete.

- Natural Killer cells, another type of lymphocyte, look for cells that lack surface markers identifying them as "self" cells and then kill them. Natural Killer cells are vital for the early immune response and the battle against cancer.

- Cells in the immune system communicate with one another via a variety of means, including the use of cytokines.

- After battling a pathogen, the immune system develops a memory for it via two routes, both of which protect the body from re-infection. The outcome is called *immunity*.

- Th2 (antibody-mediated) immunity involves the generation of antibodies by B-cells to protect against extra-cellular threats like free-floating viruses and bacteria.

- Th1 (cell-mediated) immunity involves the creation of transfer factors by Helper T-cells and the activation of Cytotoxic T-cells and Natural Killer cells to protect against intra-cellular threats like viruses, mycobacteria and CWD-bacteria that climb inside self cells.
- Transfer factors, like antibodies, bind to antigens. Unlike antibodies, transfer factors bind to antigens on the surface of infected self cells rather than on free-floating pathogens.

Now that we have covered immune system basics, we will examine the logical importance of creating and maintaining a healthy immune system. As we will see, even in those not suffering from disease states, immune system activity can strongly influence their feelings of health and well-being. In those with developmental disorders and other neuropsychiatric conditions, like depression, immune activity could play big roles.

The next three pages contain summary information related to concepts covered in Chapter 1. Along with a glossary of important terms, simple depictions of the processes leading to Th1 and Th2 immunity are provided. Though imperfect, the Th1/Th2 categorization is quite helpful for sorting out the basic mechanisms by which the body fights infections and understanding how transfer factors can help.

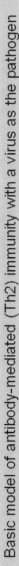

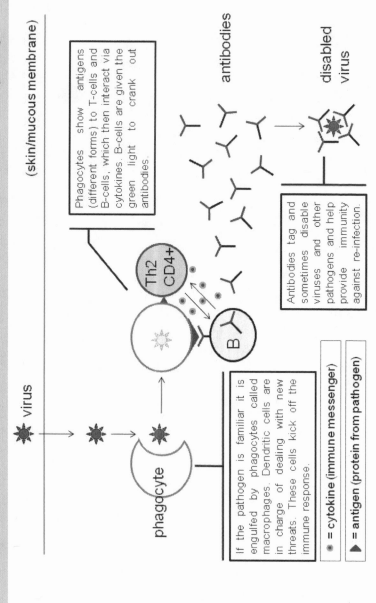

Basic model of antibody-mediated (Th2) immunity with a virus as the pathogen

(skin/mucous membrane)

virus

phagocyte

If the pathogen is familiar it is engulfed by phagocytes called macrophages. Dendritic cells are in charge of dealing with new threats. These cells kick off the immune response.

Phagocytes show antigens (different forms) to T-cells and B-cells, which then interact via cytokines. B-cells are given the green light to crank out antibodies.

Th2 CD4+

B

antibodies

Antibodies tag and sometimes disable viruses and other pathogens and help provide immunity against re-infection.

disabled virus

= cytokine (immune messenger)

= antigen (protein from pathogen)

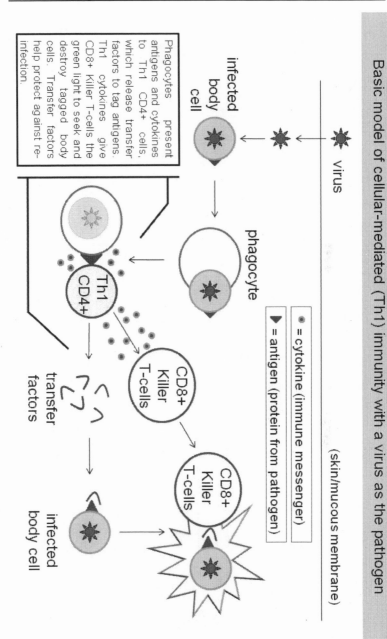

Basic model of cellular-mediated (Th1) immunity with a virus as the pathogen

virus

(skin/mucous membrane)

● = cytokine (immune messenger)

▼ = antigen (protein from pathogen)

infected body cell

phagocyte

Th1 CD4+

CD8+ Killer T-cells

CD8+ Killer T-cells

transfer factors

infected body cell

Phagocytes present antigens and cytokines to Th1 CD4+ cells, which release transfer factors to tag antigens. Th1 cytokines give CD8+ Killer T-cells the green light to seek and destroy tagged body cells. Transfer factors help protect against re-infection.

47

Glossary of important terms from Chapter 1

Pathogen	Disease causing agent, such as a virus or bacterium.
Antigen	Molecule that triggers an immune response. Often a protein on a pathogen or a body cell infected with one. Could also be a protein on a mutant cell like a cancer cell. Can also be allergens like dust, pollen or pet dander.
Antibody	Molecule made by B-cells. Binds to an antigen on a free-floating pathogen, like a virus or bacteria, or to an allergen, and disables it or marks it for destruction. Autoantibodies considered by some to lead the body to attack itself.
Helper T-cells	CD4+ cells. Detect antigens and trigger appropriate immune response, which could be antibody generation by B-cells for extracellular pathogens or transfer factor generation by CD4+ cells for intracellular infections.
Cytotoxic T-cells	CD8+ cells. Detect antigens on infected cells and directly kill the infected cells expressing them.
Natural Killer cells	Kill any cell that does not identify itself as friendly. Important in fighting cancers.
Phagocytes	Includes macrophages and dendritic cells. Gobble up pathogens and show the pathogens' antigens to other cells.
B-cells	Immune cells that make antibodies. Involved in allergies and humoral or antibody-mediated immunity. Also make the autoantibodies long thought to be responsible for autoimmune conditions, though this view is changing.
Th1 response	Immune response involving Th1 Helper T-cells, Natural Killer cells and Cytotoxic T-cells that go after body cells infected with bacteria or viruses, as well as cancer cells, fungi and protozoa. Pathway to cell-mediated immunity. Suppressed or insufficient in people with some conditions and infections, like Lyme, HIV and some autoimmune diseases.
Th2 response	Dominated by activity of Th2 Helper T-cells, B-cells and antibodies. Pathway to humoral or antibody-mediated immunity. Overactivity involved in allergies and some autoimmune conditions. Response primarily evoked by vaccines.
Transfer factor	Released by CD4+ cells. Signal CD4+ cells to direct resources toward Th1 response. Most likely help CD8+ cells identify infected host cells to destroy. Like antibodies, they bind to antigens, but on the surface of infected body cells rather than on free-floating pathogens. Small enough to be absorbed orally. Can transfer immune information from one person or other animal to another. Their importance for disease treatment and prevention could be on par with antibiotics and vaccines.

Chapter 2

The importance of a healthy immune system

The immune system comprises a complicated collection of cell types capable of working together to protect the body from foreign threats and cancer cells. Creating and maintaining a healthy immune system before disease states result is our best hope for preventing, slowing, or surviving infections of all kinds. In this chapter, we will explore the importance of creating and maintaining a healthy immune system and discuss ways in which to do so.

2.1 Reasons for creating and maintaining a healthy immune system

The flu pandemic of 1918 offers plenty of good reasons for trying to maintain a healthy immune system. In 1918 and 1919, the world was ravaged by a swine flu virus. Sometimes called the Spanish flu, the strain is now thought to have emerged in the United States. It was passed around by military personnel before being unleashed on the public. American soldiers carried it with them to Europe during WWI, where it spread like a plague through both axis and allied forces. Before burning itself out in 1919, the virus killed between 20 and 100 million people worldwide – 700,000 here in the U.S.

The good news is that not everyone infected with the virus died, just like many people, around 50%, survive the dreaded H5N1 strain of the bird flu that emerged in southern China in the mid-1990s and most (>90%) survive the H1N1 strain of swine flu that emerged in Mexico in early 2009. It is impossible to know why some people live and some do not, but keeping your immune system prepared certainly cannot hurt your odds.

In addition to decreasing the chances of contracting new diseases and dying from many existing ones, maintaining a healthy immune system can also keep old disease-causing-pathogens from flaring up. The herpes virus that causes cold sores, for instance.

Cold sores do not really have anything to do with cold viruses. They are caused by one of the many herpes viruses, Herpes Simplex Virus 1 (HSV-1). How and why would HSV-1 affect a person when they are sick with a cold? Once we contract herpes viruses, they tend to retreat inside of the nerves connecting our central nervous systems (brains and spinal cords) to the rest of our bodies. This includes the nerves that carry information to and from the face and the brain. Every now and then, for a reason usually associated with stress or an overwhelmed immune system, the herpes virus comes out of the nerves, enters skin cells and then causes them to erupt. In the case of HSV-1, the eruptions tend to occur in and around the mouth and nose. If the immune system is busy fighting another pathogen, like a cold virus, disease causing agents like HSV-1 can come out of hiding and wreak havoc. So, while not caused by a cold virus, having a cold increases the odds that opportunistic viruses, like HSV-1, will make a comeback when one is already ill.

Having a strong immune system is the best deterrent to an outbreak of viruses of all kinds, HSV-1 included. If the immune system is not working correctly, either because drugs are suppressing it, it is tied up fighting an existing illness, or because it is simply unhealthy, we become more susceptible to foreign invaders, dormant infections and cancer cells. We will return to a discussion of herpes viruses, and the potential utility of transfer factors in keeping them at bay, in a subsequent chapter.

2.2 How to avoid getting sick the old fashioned way—Flu as an example

A healthy immune system is needed to protect the body from the ravages of disease-causing viruses. Unfortunately, even the healthiest of us are susceptible to new viruses for which we lack an appropriate defense. As discussed in the previous chapter, the antigens on some viruses, like flu, mutate quickly, making it impossible for the body to be mount a rapid defense against all new strains. Indeed, one of the main fears among health officials is that a new, extremely deadly, strain of flu might emerge and quickly sweep across the globe.

In addition to actively maintaining a healthy immune system, this is where the basics, like hand washing and avoiding exposure to pathogens, come in. Below is an excerpt from a 2006 report from the World Health Organization, called "Non-pharmaceutical interventions for pandemic influenza, international measures" (WHO, 2006).

> "Pandemic preparedness ideally would include pharmaceutical countermeasures (vaccine and antiviral drugs), but for the foreseeable future, such measures will not be available for the global population of >6 billion. Thus, in 2005… the

World Health Organization (WHO) recommended nonpharmaceutical public health interventions in its updated global influenza preparedness plans. Such interventions, designed to reduce exposure of susceptible persons to an infectious agent, were commonly used for infection control in previous centuries."

Frequent hand washing and avoiding contact with sick people are powerful approaches to escaping the flu. Again, having a healthy immune system also helps. According to the CDC (same article as above):

"Serologic testing indicates that approximately 30%-50% of seasonal influenza infections may not result in illness".

There must be something about some exposed people that allows them to beat the virus early before it creates a problem. Of course, we are talking about the typical flu bug here, not the supervirus that world health officials now fear.

There are limits to how well we can protect ourselves. The common flu virus can be spread by infected persons 24-48 hrs before symptoms emerge. A closed-door business meeting could lead to a rapid spread of the illness before anyone even becomes ill. According to the CDC (again, same article as above):

"Influenzalike illness developed in 72% of passengers seated in an airplane that was on the ground for 3 h without ventilation and that held a person with symptomatic influenza. On a 75-seat aircraft, 15 passengers traveling with an influenza-infected person became ill. All 15 persons were seated within 5 rows of the index patient, and 9 were seated within 2 rows."

Because there are limits to how well the immune system can protect us from highly contagious pathogens, the best gift we can give ourselves, and our communities, when we have the flu — whether the seasonal variety or a pandemic superbug — is to stay home. According to a recent report by Michael Haber from Emory University and colleagues from the CDC (Haber et al, 2007):

"..if persons with influenzalike symptoms and their household contacts were encouraged to stay home, then rates of illness and death might be reduced by $\approx 50\%$."

And, so, despite the lack of magic pharmaceutical bullets to prevent viral pandemics, low-tech strategies like hand washing and avoiding contact with sick people, along with maintaining a healthy immune system, remain quite effective.

2.3 Heart disease and immune system health – Could viruses and bacteria cause heart problems and stroke?

Yes. According to recent information from the American Heart Association, infectious diseases could be the culprits underlying heart disease and strokes in many people:

"No one knows for sure what causes the low-grade inflammation that seems to put otherwise healthy people at risk. However, the new findings are consistent with the hypothesis that an infection – possibly one caused by a bacteria or a virus – might contribute to or even cause atherosclerosis. Possible infectious bacteria include Chlamydia pneumoniae (klah-MID'e-ah nu-MO'ne-i) and Helicobacter pylori (HEL'ih-ko-bak"ter pi-LO'ri). Possible viral agents include herpes simplex virus and cytomegalovirus (si"to-meg"ah-lo-VI'rus). Thus, it may be that antimicrobial or antiviral therapies will someday join other therapies used to prevent heart attacks."

See AHA, 2007 in the references for a link to the full article. Keep in mind that other factors, like stress, also play contributing roles in heart attack and stroke, and infections are unlikely to explain all cases. However, the link between heart disease, stroke and infections highlights the central role that the immune system seems to play in a very wide range of health conditions.

2.4 Immune system health and well-being

Research has begun to elucidate the relationship between immune system health and general feelings of well-being. Researchers in Israel examined the psychological well-being of teenage girls vaccinated for the rubella virus, a common cause of illness in kids. As discussed previously, vaccination involves injecting portions of a virus, or even the whole virus, into the body so that the immune system can learn to recognize it and protect the person from the virus if ever encountered in the real world. Following vaccinations, the immune system becomes acutely active as it learns about the antigens, making some people feel ill. In the aforementioned study, those that became slightly ill also became slightly depressed. In the words of the author (Yirmaya, 2000):

"[Some of the vaccinated girls] showed a significant rise in several standard measures of depressed mood, as well as an increased incidence of social and attention problems and delinquent behavior... Thus, even a mild viral infection can produce a prolonged increase in depressive symptoms in vulnerable persons."

The same group of researchers took their investigations into the relationship between immune system health and psychological functioning one step further. They injected small portions of the cell walls from bacteria into subjects, a technique commonly used to evoke an immune response in humans in order to assess immune system function. Even though the injected material caused no physical symptoms,

"The subjects showed a transient substantial increase in levels of anxiety and depressed mood. In addition, verbal and nonverbal memory functions were substantially impaired."

In another study of mood in young females after rubella vaccination, the researchers found similar results (Yirmaya et al, 2000):

"Compared to control group subjects and to their own baseline, a subgroup of vulnerable individuals (girls from low socioeconomic status) showed a significant virus-induced increase in depressed mood up to 10 weeks after vaccination."

Similar outcomes occur when subjects are injected with cytokines, molecules released as part of the body's immune response. Researchers at the University of Illinois Champagne-Urbana argue that cytokines cause many of the psychological symptoms of illness by acting directly in the brain. Here's what they had to say in a recent paper (Dantzer and Kelley, 2006):

> Cytokines "act in the brain to induce common symptoms of sickness, such as loss of appetite, sleepiness, withdrawal from normal social activities, fever, aching joints and fatigue…The fact that cytokines act in the brain to induce physiological adaptations that promote survival has led to the hypothesis that inappropriate, prolonged activation of the innate immune system may be involved in a number of pathological disturbances in the brain, ranging from Alzheimer's disease to stroke…Indeed, the newest findings of cytokine actions in the brain offer some of the first clues about the pathophysiology of certain mental health disorders, including depression."

Interestingly, antidepressants suppress production of some cytokines and have been found to reduce the symptoms of cytokine-induced depression (Nishidaa et al., 2002). Exercise, which is roughly equal in efficacy to pharmaceutical drugs against depression, also produces robust changes in immune system health, stimulating the production of Natural Killer cells even after a single, 90 minute session of moderate exertion. Thus, both exercise and antidepressants could exert effects on mood via influences on the immune system.

Immune system activity affects how we feel and how we feel affects immune system activity. Researchers at the Indiana State School of Nursing reported that having cancer patients view humorous programs leads to increases in Natural Killer cell levels. In their words (Bennett et al, 2003):

"Laughter may reduce stress and improve NK cell activity. As low NK cell activity is linked to decreased disease resistance and increased morbidity in persons with cancer and HIV disease, laughter may be a useful cognitive-behavioral intervention."

Thus, it appears that activity within the immune system can have a big impact on how otherwise healthy people think and feel. And feeling well promotes immune system health. Additional reasons to work hard at maintaining a healthy immune system.

2.5 The role of the immune system in psychiatric conditions and developmental disorders

As detailed above, activity in the immune system can influence levels of anxiety and depressive symptoms in otherwise mentally healthy people. Researchers have long speculated that there are also links between immune system health and psychiatric conditions. Studies performed decades ago suggested that exposure to certain strains of the flu virus during the third trimester of pregnancy could influence the likelihood that offspring would develop schizophrenia. More recent studies have begun to link psychiatric conditions with specific types of infections and immune imbalances.

A new category of pediatric ailments called Pediatric Autoimmune Neuropsychiatric Disorders Associated with Streptococcal infections (PANDAS) highlights the strong ties between immune activity and psychological functioning. Symptoms of PANDAS include sudden onset tick disorders and obsessive compulsive disorder and are thought to be caused by an autoimmune reaction. It appears that immune cells seeking the strep bacteria might attack brain cells in an area called the basal ganglia. The basal ganglia are involved in voluntary movement, timing, planning sequences of movements, anxiety and emotional – usually fearful – reactions to stimuli. When these structures are inflamed and under attack, a whole host of psychological symptoms emerges. Whether the cells in the basal ganglia are infected or the attack is truly autoimmune (i.e., unprovoked) is unclear.

Researchers believe that one variant of transfer factor molecules activates Suppressor T-cells and calms autoimmune responses. It is therefore possible that transfer factors could be engineered to help balance the immune system in children with PANDAS and calm the autoimmune response, perhaps leading to a diminution of symptoms. If the condition is triggered by intracellular pathogens, transfer factors could help solve the underlying problem. On a positive note, current thinking holds that many children with PANDAS age out of the condition, perhaps as the immune system matures.

Sperner-Unterweger (2005) summarizes the link between immune system health and psychiatric conditions as follows:

> "Treatment strategies based on immune mechanisms have been investigated in patients with schizophrenia and affective disorders. Furthermore, some antipsychotics and most antidepressants are known to have direct or indirect effects on the immune system. Different immunotherapies have been used in autism, including transfer factor, pentoxifylline, intravenous immunoglobulins and corticosteroids. Immunosuppressive and/or immunomodulating agents are well established methods for treating the neuropsychiatric sequelae of immune or autoimmune disorders, for example AIDS and SLE. Therapeutic approaches in

Alzheimer's disease also apply immunological methods such as strategies of active/passive immunisation and NSAIDs. Considering the comprehensive interactive network between mind and body, future research should focus on approaches linking targets of the different involved systems."

And with regard to the etiology and treatment of autism, a debilitating neurocognitive disorder on the rise, Kidd (2002) tells us:

"Autism and allied autistic spectrum disorders (ASD) present myriad behavioral, clinical, and biochemical abnormalities... Immune therapies (pentoxifyllin, intravenous immunoglobulin, transfer factor, and colostrum) benefit selected cases... Current pharmaceuticals fail to benefit the primary symptoms and can have marked adverse effects. Individualized, in-depth clinical and laboratory assessments and integrative parent-physician-scientist cooperation are the keys to successful ASD management."

An immune system link would certainly help explain the increasing rates of autism. According to the Autism Society of America (www.autism-society.org), rates of the disorder are growing at roughly 10-17% per year. An article in the Sacramento Bee (Whitney, 2003) reports that researchers at UC-Davis estimated in 2003 that California was:

"...adding an average of 11 names a day to its list of severely autistic children qualifying for state-financed services. The average lifetime cost of these educational services is $4 million per child. As a result, the increase in children eligible for services represents an increase in the state's long-term financial responsibility of $44 million a day."

Dozens of studies published during the past few years support an immune-link for autism. In particular, heightened immune activity in the brain early in life is thought to be involved (Pardo et al, 2005). Regardless of the underlying culprit, Cohly and Panja (2005) suggest that, in some patients, the result is the following:

> "Cell-mediated immunity is impaired as evidenced by low numbers of CD4 cells and a concomitant T-cell polarity with an imbalance of Th1/Th2 subsets toward Th2."

This begins to make autism look like an autoimmune condition, meaning it could involve an intracellular infection or an aberrant immune response aimed at ultimately healthy cells.

In the 3rd edition of her informative book, *Children with Starving Brains: A Medical Treatment Guide for Autism Spectrum Disorder*, Dr. Jaquelyn McCandless notes several common immune issues in autistic children, including:

- Low numbers of Helper T-cells
- Decreased Natural Killer cell function
- Depressed T-cell responses to activation

Speculation regarding the cause of these immune abnormalities has included viral infections and the measles-mumps-rubella (MMR) vaccine. The relationship, if any, between MMR vaccination and autism is an issue that would require a full book to unravel and the evidence will not be reviewed here. In summary, the link is tenuous. However, there seem to be legitimate reasons to suspect that vaccines could have serious health consequences for a small percentage of kids. Historically, vaccines have been linked with autoimmune conditions in some recipients. The 1976 H1N1 (swine flu) vaccine was associated with an estimated 500 cases of the autoimmune condition, Guillain-Barré syndrome. The vaccine approach is geared toward evoking antibody production and a strong Th2 response (see Page 25 for discussion). This can have repercussions – physically and psychologically.

New research suggests that heightened antibody-mediated immunity in pregnant moms could be the culprit in some cases of autism. In 2008, researchers at UC Davis reported that the immune systems of mothers of autistic children contain antibodies that bind to proteins in fetal brain cells, raising the possibility that hyperactive antibody-mediated immune activity in pregnant women could impact fetal brain development leading to autism. Alternatively, antibodies against fetal brain proteins could indicate the presence of intracellular infections of some sort in fetal brain cells. Findings similar to those from UC Davis were reported by doctors at Johns Hopkins that same year.

It is possible that vaccines influence the risk of autism through their effects on the *mother's*, rather than the *child's*, immune system. During pregnancy, the balance of immune function naturally tilts in the Th2 direction, presumably because a strong Th1 response could lead the body to reject the baby as in cases of organ transplants. If the mother's immune system is already tilted too far in the Th2 direction, perhaps due to lingering effects of childhood vaccinations or the presence of autoimmune conditions, this could spell trouble and might explain the generation of autoantibodies to fetal brain cell proteins. Indeed, autoimmune conditions are quite common in mothers of autistic children, occurring in 30% or more.

Immune system dysfunction – including both Th1 and Th2 hyperactivity – is also associated with psychopathologies such as depression. Ranga Krishnan and colleagues at Duke University Medical Center (Suarez et al, 2003) measured levels of depression and markers of proinflammatory cytokines from blood samples drawn from healthy young men. Even those with moderate levels of depressive symptoms exhibited higher levels of Th1-related proinflammatory immune markers.

Depression is associated with cardiovascular disease. Krishnan and colleagues suggest the link between depression and cardiovascular disease could be mitigated through high levels of Th1 proinflammatory cytokines, including tumor necrosis factor (TNF), which is also associated with autoimmune conditions like rheumatoid arthritis and psoriasis.

If depression is linked to inflammation, the direction of the relationship might run both ways. That is, proinflammatory cytokines, perhaps related to an infection, trigger negative emotional changes. The resulting emotional changes, including depression, increase levels of proinflammatory cytokines.

Bipolar depression is yet another condition linked to immune health. Bipolar depression often follows a course reminiscent of recurrent viral outbreaks. The possibility of a link between bipolar and the immune system is strengthened by the observation that lithium, one of the most effective treatments for the condition, has potent antiviral and immunomodulatory effects. Amsterdam et al (1990) and Rybakowski (2000) report that lithium reduces the symptoms of bipolar and also reduces the frequency of herpes outbreaks in infected bipolar patients.

In summary, immune activity is related to psychological well-being. Mild ailments can cause transient increases in depression and anxiety. Chronic conditions often bring chronic issues with affect. Immune dysfunction plays a role in autism, but it remains unclear what that role is. It could be related to Th2 hyperimmunity in the mother or perhaps to intracellular infections in fetal brain cells. Inflammation caused by Th1 hyperactivity is related to depression and could explain the link between depression and cardiovascular disease. Some of the benefits of psychotherapeutic medications, such as antidepressants, could stem from their effects on both Th1 and Th2 activity in the immune system.

2.6 Healthy immune systems require more than meds – Sunlight and Vitamin D as examples

Maintaining a healthy immune system is an active process. Exercise, supplements, and some drugs can help, but there are also some very basic needs that must be met if one is to remain healthy. One of those basic needs is exposure to the sun.

Most cells in the body contain receptors for Vitamin D. Not surprisingly, this vitamin plays several vital roles in health. These include providing calcium to bones and reducing the likelihood that healthy cells will become cancerous. Vitamin D plays a variety of roles in immune system functioning. Vitamin D deficiencies are hypothesized by some to contribute to the pathophysiology underlying autoimmune conditions like MS and the development of cancers. Others believe the problems are related to levels of Vitamin D that are too high.

Sunlight is central to Vitamin D production. The vitamin is produced by the skin in response to being bombarded with quanta of UV light from the sun. Researchers estimate that 90% of the Vitamin D our bodies need is generated by exposure to sunlight. Australian researchers estimate that fair skinned Australians need between 2-14 minutes of exposure to midday sun three-four times per week with 15% of their skin exposed to generate a sufficient amount of the vitamin (Samanek et al, 2006). Necessary exposure times are longer for people with darker skin.

Too little exposure to sunlight serves as a risk factor in the development of MS, presumably because of the reduced Vitamin D production. In twins in which one has MS and the other does not, the one who spends more time in the sun is less likely to develop the disorder.

Exposure to sunlight is critical for immune system health beyond Vitamin D production. Exposure to either the sun or broad spectrum light activates the immune system and increases white blood cell counts in healthy people. Both sunlight and Vitamin D supplementation have been found to boost mood and ease depression. One half hour per morning of broad spectrum 10,000 lux light has been found to alleviate symptoms of Seasonal Affective Disorder.

In short, despite the fact that we humans have learned to function at any time of the day or night, and that we have developed supplements and drugs capable of boosting immune system health, exposure to sunlight remains central to our basic physiological health, from the single cell on up.

2.7 Breastfeeding and childhood health – The immune system link

Given the fact that colostrum, and then normal breast milk after it, contains vital immune information, it might not surprise the reader to learn that questions have been raised about the link between breast feeding, more specifically the lack thereof, and childhood illnesses.

In a fascinating review of the literature on breastfeeding and public health, published in the *American Journal of Public Health*, Dr. Jacqueline Wolf from Ohio University makes a compelling argument that breastfeeding is far better for kids than formula when it comes to promoting health (Wolf, 2003):

> "...contemporary research demonstrates that exclusive breastfeeding for 6 months and pro-longed breastfeeding thereafter is key to main-

taining children's and women's health. Extended breastfeeding not only reduces the incidence in children of acute illnesses such as diarrhea, ear infections, pneumonia, and meningitis, it lessens the occurrence of chronic diseases and conditions such as sudden infant death syndrome (SIDS), obesity, childhood leukemia, asthma, and lowered IQ. And women who practice prolonged breastfeeding enjoy significantly reduced rates of breast cancer."

She reminds the reader that this is not the first time we have dealt with this problem in our culture. According to Dr. Wolf, in the early part of the 20th century, public health officials posted signs saying,

"To lessen baby deaths let us have more mother-fed babies. You can't improve on God's plan. For your baby's sake – nurse it!"

The website for Enfamil, made by Mead Johnson Nutritionals (see Enfamil, 2007 in references for link), details some of the discrepancies between formula and real breast milk. The company lists important improvements in its breast milk formulas over the years (see the next page). Given that science is still working to identify the important constituents of breast milk, there is little doubt that key ingredients are still absent.

In 2005, Mead Johnson announced that they were the first formula maker to increase levels of dietary choline to the levels found in breast milk. This is probably good news for kids. Among other things, choline is the precursor for acetylcholine – a brain chemical that plays important roles in learning, memory and attention.

"Approaching the Gold Standard: Breast Milk

In the 1980s and '90s, more advances brought Enfamil even closer to breast milk:

- In 1981, the protein content was modified to be less like cow's milk and more like breast milk, offering a whey-to-casein ratio of 60:40. Just like breast milk.
- In 1992, the fat blend was reformulated again, getting even closer to breast milk.
- In 1996, free nucleotides (building blocks of DNA and RNA) were added at the level found in breast milk.
- In 2002, Enfamil with Iron included LIPIL, a blend of DHA and ARA, important nutrients found in breast milk that support brain and eye development.
- By mid-year 2003, LIPIL had been added to most of the Enfamil Family of Formulas™."

(From www.enfamil.com)

A few years ago, the author of the current book worked with Scott Swartzwelder at Duke University Medical Center on a study in which pregnant rats were given extra choline in their diets and the effects of the choline on brain function in the offspring were measured (Li et al, 2004). It is known that the offspring of rats fed extra choline during pregnancy learn maze tasks faster than their peers later in life. In this study, we observed that cells in memory-related brain circuits in the hippocampus are larger and function better in the offspring of high-choline moms. This could explain why the offspring of high-choline moms learn so fast and highlights the importance of proper nutrition early in life for healthy development.

That project, along with several conducted by researchers like Steve Zeisel at UNC Chapel Hill (see Zeisel, 2004 for review) highlight the importance of early exposure to the nutrient choline for later development. Breast milk is a rich source of choline and many other critical nutrients. It is entirely possible that formula could one day be superior to breast milk, but it will likely be a while. This is not due to a lack of effort on the part of formula makers. The problem is that we know so little about what kids really need early in life, in terms of nutrition. Because some of those issues are yet to be resolved, breast milk remains more complete than formulas for obvious reasons.

The Center for Science in the Public Interest (CSPI) provides a sobering critique of the oversight of formula production. In a review of how the FDA regulates product contents, product labeling, quality control and other issues, CSPI states the following with regard to formula (Heller et al, 2003):

> "The Infant Formula Act of 1980 sets minimum and maximum levels of specified nutrients for formulas. FDA may revise the list. The Agency is also authorized to establish quality control requirements for infant formula and must oversee product recalls. On July 9, 1996, FDA issued a proposed rule to establish requirements for current good manufacturing practices and audits, establish requirements for quality factors, and amend its quality control procedures, notification, and records and reports requirements. Nearly seven years later, FDA reopened the comment period to receive new information. While this rulemaking was pending, there was an outbreak of E. Sakazaki among 10 infants in a Tennessee Hospital. One of them died."

It seems appropriate to let Dr. Wolf have the last word in this section (Wolf, 2004):

> "Feeding babies should be a risk-free venture, which is why the American propensity to for-

mula-feed is so troubling. We need to solve this international public health problem. However, limiting infants' exposure to human milk is no solution."

2.8 Summary

A healthy immune system is critical for preventing and overcoming ailments of all kinds. When exposed to pathogens like viruses and bacteria, a prompt and healthy immune response can minimize the number of days spent sick and could potentially make the difference between life and death. Doing what we can to maximize our immune system health could minimize the likelihood that we will contract, and perhaps subsequently spread, diseases.

The health of the immune system has a powerful impact on the general quality of an individual's life. This is obvious to those who are ill, but perhaps less obvious to those who are not. Research strongly suggests that even subtle changes in immune system activity, such as changes following vaccinations, can directly impact our emotional well-being, perhaps via the effects of cytokines on activity in the brain.

Armed with background material on basic immune system functioning and the importance of creating and maintaining a healthy immune system, we will now turn our attention to a fascinating type of immune messenger called transfer factors. As we will see, transfer factors are capable of directly influencing the health and functioning of the immune system in profound ways and could have enormous potential for the treatment and prevention of infectious diseases and other immune conditions in the 21st century.

Chapter 3

Transfer factors – What they are and how they work

Transfer factor (TF)...has been used successfully over the past quarter of a century for treating viral, parasitic, and fungal infections, as well as immunodeficiencies, neoplasias, allergies and autoimmune diseases. Moreover, several observations suggest that it can be utilized for prevention, transferring immunity prior to infection...Thus, a specific TF to a new influenza virus can be made swiftly and used for prevention as well as for the treatment of infected patients.

- Giancarlo Pizza et al, 2006

The human body provides a lucrative environment for bacteria, viruses and other pathogens. Some can be beaten by healthy immune systems alone while others require external treatment in the form of medicine, modified diets and so on.

Fortunately, the last century witnessed several important advances in disease treatment and prevention. Antibiotics, discovered in the 1920s, proved to be lifesavers against bacterial infections. Vaccines became widely used in the 20th century for disease prevention. The undeniable success of antibiotics for treating bacterial infections and vaccines for preventing bacterial and viral infections overshadowed the importance of a third development – the discovery of transfer factors – in the late 1940s.

In this chapter, we will explore the discovery of transfer factors and what is known regarding their structure and function. To place their discovery and their potential importance for medicine and public health in context we will begin by examining the discovery of antibiotics and the development of vaccines. As we will see, transfer factors can help fill gaps in disease treatment and prevention left by these approaches.

3.1 The discovery of antibiotics and the reign of vaccines in the 20th century

In 1928, in a laboratory in London, Alexander Fleming observed that a common species of mold known as Penicillium was capable of killing bacteria in Petri dishes. He was not the first to notice the bacteria-killing properties of Penicillium, but neither Dr. Fleming nor the rest of the world were aware of the original discovery made by a French medical student in 1896. By all accounts, Dr. Fleming did not intend to discover an antibiotic. He returned to his lab after some time away and found that the bacteria he was culturing did not grow within a narrow zone around the fringes of an annoying mold that contaminated his samples. Dr. Fleming identified the component of the mold with antibacterial properties and labeled it, "penicillin". It would be more than a decade – during the late 1930s – before researchers realized the full potential of penicillin and figured out how to turn Dr. Fleming's discovery into a mass producible treatment for disease. Widespread use of antibiotics began in the 1940s and 50s, thus ushering in an era in which rates of death due to infections and communicable bacteria plummeted.

Vaccines, discovered centuries earlier, had an equally dramatic impact on the spread of disease in the mid-20th century. While antibiotics were wiping out one bacterial infection after another, vaccines for preventing the spread of infectious diseases were developed at a rapid pace. Six vaccines were in the arsenal prior to the 1900s. By 1970, 14 more had been added with varying degrees of success – including vaccines for tuberculosis (1927), typhus (1937), influenza (1945), polio (1952), measles (1963), mumps (1967) and rubella (1970). Thus, the 20th century truly was an era of miraculous developments in medicine.

3.2 The discovery of transfer factors and their potential to reshape medicine in the 21st century

In 1949, at a time when the benefits of vaccines were becoming apparent and penicillin, along with the sulfa antibiotics developed in Germany, were gaining reputations as wonder drugs, a tuberculosis researcher named Dr. H Sherwood Lawrence made another important discovery in disease treatment and prevention. He extracted intracellular fluid from circulating white blood cells in patients who had been exposed to tuberculosis (TB). He then injected the contents of these cells into non-exposed patients. Using a test for an immune response known as Delayed Type Hypersensitivity, he demonstrated that the non-exposed patient's immune system now recognized TB and responded to it as though it had already fought it. In other words, immunity to TB was somehow *transferred* from one person to the next via the white blood cell extract.

Dr. Lawrence referred to the contents of the white blood cells from the host as Dialyzable Leukocyte Extract, because the fluid was extracted from white blood cells (leukocytes) and then filtered to get rid of large particles (dialysis). In the years that followed, Dr. Lawrence began to refer to the mystery components within the Dialyzable Leukocyte Extract as "transfer factor," as they somehow transferred immunity from one patient to the next. Dr. Lawrence was already a seasoned researcher in immunology. His excitement at the initial discovery must have been an experience akin to other "Eureka!" moments in science.

Research during the decades since suggests that the information contained in the molecules Dr. Lawrence called transfer factor can instruct the immune system to do several different things, thus transferring immunity via different routes, and might actually come in several – three to be exact – basic sizes. Thus, rather than one factor, there seem to be multiple factors involved in transferring immunity. For this reason, the plural transfer factors is used throughout this book.

3.3 Where do transfer factors come from, why are they made, and how do they work?

Transfer factors are relatively short chains of amino acids and, it appears, RNA. Their exact length and make up are not known for certain, but an estimate from researchers holding a patent for the extraction of transfer factors from colostrum and egg yolk places their length at roughly 45 amino acids divided into three sections (Hennen and Lisonbee, 2002). One section binds to pathogens. One section binds to T-cells. The third area is a connector region between the first two. The role played by the RNA, if in fact present, remains unstudied, but could be used to influence gene expression in T-cells, leading to the changes in cytokine release and Natural Killer cell levels that follow transfer factor therapy.

It is believed that transfer factors are created inside of Helper T-cells, also known as CD4+ cells. These cells contain special receptors on their surfaces to which a specific antigen can bind, thereby triggering a chain of events that leads to a full-blown immune response to the pathogen expressing the antigen. Each Helper T-cell is thought to release transfer factors capable of binding to the same antigen to which the Helper T-cell binds. It is possible that transfer factors are free-floating copies of the antigen receptors present on Helper T-cells but this remains unknown (Kirkpatrick and Rozzo, 1995).

It appears that Helper T-cells contain special binding sites for one part of transfer factor molecules. In 2000, Dr. Charles Kirkpatrick and his colleagues identified a conserved amino acid sequence in transfer factors, meaning that all transfer factors seem to contain this particular strand of amino acids plus whatever it is that makes each one specific to a pathogen. Next, they demonstrated that administering this conserved sequence to mice receiving complete transfer factor molecules blocked the effects of the complete transfer factors, a finding similar to how some drugs shaped like neurotransmitters prevent neurotransmitters from activating their target receptors on brain cells.

Kirkpatrick believes that this conserved sequence represents the portion of the transfer factor molecule that binds to receptors on T-cells. Once bound, the remaining portion of the molecule swings into action, perhaps placing the antigen into its correct binding site on the T-cell membrane. When only the conserved sequence is administered, it blocks the ability of complete transfer factors to bind and present the antigen, thus blocking the effects of the complete transfer factors.

While Th1 Helper T-cells direct the immune response toward fighting intracellular infections, Cytotoxic T-cells do the job of hunting down infected self cells and destroying them. Like Helper T-cells, Cytotoxic T-cells contain receptors on their cell membranes for the antigen of interest. Just as transfer factors seem to facilitate binding of the antigen to Helper T-cells, it is possible they also help facilitate binding of the antigen to Cytotoxic T-cells, thereby playing an important role in helping Cytotoxic T-cells identify and destroy infected self cells.

If the above scenario is accurate, then transfer factors act in some ways like antibodies, in that both bind to specific antigens and mark the antigen-bearing object for destruction. Whereas antibodies tag free-floating viruses and bacteria, transfer factors tag self cells infected with viruses and bacteria. Transfer factors also function a bit like immune system enzymes, sticking T-cells and infected cells together.

It is possible that transfer factors influence key aspects of immune function by triggering Th1-related immune cells to release cytokines, thereby influencing immune activity down-stream. Kirkpatrick's research suggests this is the case. He and his colleagues measured levels of various cytokines following the oral administration of transfer factors to human subjects. Of the cytokines, only levels of gamma-interferon (INFγ) increased. Why is that interesting? INFγ is only produced by Type 1 Helper T-cells (Th1), Cytotoxic T-cells and Natural Killer cells, thus indicating the specificity of transfer factors for activating the Th1 response pathway. INFγ is an important and powerful cytokine. It can disable viruses and kill cancer cells. It can also cause young white blood cells to differentiate into Th1 cells, perhaps partially explaining how transfer factors lead to the recruitment of new cells for Th1 immune battles.

While synthetic INFγ is used in the treatment of certain disease states, like hepatitis C, its poor side effect profile and subtle differences between synthetic INFγ and human-made INFγ make it less than ideal. Whether the INFγ production triggered by transfer factors is sufficient to replace the synthetic sources of INFγ is currently unknown.

3.4 Immunity conveyed by transfer factors

Transfer factor, now commonly used in the plural, was so named because of its ability to transfer cell-mediated immunity from a previously – or currently – infected patient to a naïve one. This is commonly demonstrated using a Delayed Hypersensitivity Test in which a person has a small amount of the pathogen, or a portion of it, placed into the skin via a pin prick. If the individual has already been exposed to that pathogen, and the immune system works correctly, macrophages engulf the pathogen and then present the antigen associated with the pathogen to Helper T-cells and Cytotoxic T-cells. These cells then release cytokines to coordinate additional components of the Th1 immune response. Redness and swelling related to this cell-mediated immune response can be observed at the contact site within 24-72 hours, hence the designation "delayed hypersensitivity". If the individual has not been exposed to the pathogen, some redness and swelling occur early on but the delayed reaction is not present.

A real world example of delayed hypersensitivity involves exposure to poison ivy, in which itching and irritation develop to the toxin over a period of hours or days.

A naïve person (one that does not exhibit delayed hypersensitivity to a pathogen) given transfer factors taken from a previously exposed host (one that does exhibit delayed hypersensitivity to the pathogen) will subsequently display delayed hypersensitivity to the pathogen. In other words, the transfer factors somehow transfer cell-mediated immunity from the exposed host to the naïve host.

In order for this to occur, transfer factors must somehow educate the individual's naïve immune system about the pathogen and then stimulate the generation of T-cells and other immune cells capable of responding to the pathogen once it enters the body. From a practical standpoint, it is as if the memory of previous immune battles is contained in the small molecules that comprise transfer factors, and that the code can be passed on from person to person, saving non-exposed people the hassle of having to develop immunity the hard way.

Let us walk through a theoretical example involving the transfer of immunity to tuberculosis, as first observed by Dr. Lawrence. We begin with two patients. One patient has already been exposed to one or both of the mycobacteria that cause tuberculosis - *Mycobacterium tuberculosis* and *Mycobacterium bovis*. The other individual has not. As such, the exposed patient's Helper T-cells already contain transfer factors specific to the antigens associated with the mycobacteria. The naïve individual's Helper T-cells have not created such transfer factors. Once extracted from the intracellular fluid of Helper T-cells from the exposed individual, the Dialyzable Leukocyte Extract containing the transfer factors can be administered to the naïve individual. Transfer factors in the Dialyzable Leukocyte Extract contain all of the information necessary for the naïve host's immune system to respond quickly and aggressively to the tuberculosis mycobacteria if they ever enter the body. As such, the transfer factors allow the naïve person to become immune to tuberculosis without being exposed to the mycobacteria first. Evidence of the transmitted immunity manifests in positive tests for Delayed Type Hypersensitivity to tuberculosis in those receiving the transfer factors.

3.5 How do transfer factors differ from vaccines?

Both transfer factors and vaccines can be used to immunize people against infectious diseases. Transfer factors differ from vaccines in the process by which they help the body become immune. Transfer factors directly transfer cell-mediated immunity and prepare the host's body to quickly attack and destroy a pathogen using a Th1-mediated immune response if the pathogen enters the body. They provide the immune system with information to be used in the future and do not trigger a large-scale immune response when administered (unless of course the targeted pathogen is already present in the body).

Immunity developed through vaccination involves a different process. Portions of a pathogen, and sometimes deactivated forms of the entire pathogen, are injected into a naïve host. This process provokes B-cells to generate antibodies to antigens in the vaccine. Memory B-cells are left behind and are capable of cranking out antibodies in a hurry if the real virus or bacterium ever enters the body.

While this is where the story about vaccines usually ends, it is important to point out that, presumably, the process of vaccination sometimes triggers the creation of pathogen-specific transfer factors by Helper T-cells, at least in cases where either a live pathogen is used or a deactivated pathogen that is at least still capable of penetrating into host cells. (If a host cell displays antigens related to the pathogen on its cell membrane, it is likely that transfer factors are created as a result.) In some cases, the effectiveness of vaccines could rest in their ability to trigger both antibody-mediated *and* cell-mediated immunity, despite the tendency of many vaccines to preferentially activate antibody-mediated immunity (see Page 25 in Chapter 1 for a discussion of vaccines and antibody-mediated immunity).

Supplemental transfer factors circumvent the need for the initial immune response that leads to cell-mediated immunity. They prime the patient's immune system to respond as though it has already been down that path before. Whether transfer factors lead to the development of specific antibodies by B-cells is not known, but seems unlikely.

Transfer factors and vaccines differ in a very practical way, too. Transfer factors can be made quickly by exposing a cow or a chicken to a pathogen of interest, extracting the transfer factors from the cow colostrum or the egg yolk, and using lab techniques to isolate transfer factors specific to the antigens associated with the pathogen (Kirkpatrick and Rozzo, 1995). Transfer factors for new forms of a pathogen, like new H5N1 and H1N1 strains of the flu virus, could be made and distributed in a matter of weeks. Unlike vaccines, they can be sent through the mail and taken orally. They also appear to be incredibly safe. In contrast, vaccines are difficult and slow to make, can have dire consequences for the recipient, and most must be injected, though some can be inhaled. Let us look at the vaccine process using vaccines for flu as an example.

Flu vaccines come in two types – injectable and inhalable. Each year, researchers from around the planet convene to identify which three strains of the virus are the most likely to go around. Flu vaccines are then made by injecting the virus into fertilized chicken eggs and allowing it to replicate over the next 11 days. Vaccine production is very slow and must begin around 6-9 months before flu season. This makes it difficult for vaccine makers to plan perfectly, and essentially impossible to make a vaccine for a new strain quickly.

Because of the speed with which transfer factors can be created, they could be ideal for contending with emerging strains of flu. According to the Italian researcher Giancarlo Pizza and colleagues (2006):

> "Avian influenza…presents a threat of producing a pandemic. The consensus is that the occurrence of such a pandemic is only a matter of time. This is of great concern, since no effective vaccine is available or can be made before the occurrence of the event. We present arguments for the use of cell mediated immunity for the prevention of the infection as well as for the treatment of infected patients. Transfer factor (TF)…has been used successfully over the past quarter of a century for treating viral, parasitic, and fungal infections, as well as immunodeficiencies, neoplasias, allergies

> and autoimmune diseases. Moreover, several observations suggest that it can be utilized for prevention, transferring immunity prior to infection…Thus, a specific TF to a new influenza virus can be made swiftly and used for prevention as well as for the treatment of infected patients."

As discussed in Chapter 1, flu viruses exhibit a lot of what is called *antigenic drift*. Over time, the viruses mutate and their antigens change. Because of this antigenic drift, there is no way, at least not yet, to immunize someone against all flu viruses and new vaccines must be generated prior to each flu season. The process often leads to vaccines with poor efficacy. Indeed, in early 2009, the CDC announced that the highly touted flu vaccine Tamiflu had no effect whatsoever on that season's flu viruses. Transfer factors could prove particularly useful against viruses that exhibit a high degree of antigenic drift.

A prominent difference between transfer factors and vaccines rests in their safety profiles. Side effects from vaccines are relatively rare but can be quite serious. According to the CDC, the inhalable flu vaccine, Tamiflu, can produce a host of neuropsychiatric side effects, including nervousness and delirium (confusion), particularly in children. In Japan, where use of Tamiflu is more widespread, dozens of deaths have been associated with it, many due to apparent suicides. No such side effects have been reported in studies using transfer factors. Side effects from transfer factors seem to be limited to mild cold- or flu-like symptoms sometime early in treatment. These symptoms reflect heightened immune function and, according to reports, usually resolve within a few weeks.

As we will discuss in Chapter 6, it is unlikely that transfer factors can relegate all vaccines to the back of the medical tool shed, but they do provide a powerful, practical and safe means of immunizing people against infectious diseases. Vaccines for simple viruses like HPV, linked to cervical cancer, are ideal candidates for replacement by transfer factors. The value of transfer factors for public health could be assessed easily against viruses like hepatitis C and the noroviruses that ruin cruise ship vacations for thousands of passengers each year.

3.6 Why activating the immune system with transfer factors can calm some autoimmune conditions

Autoimmune conditions have long been considered conditions in which an over-eager immune system attacks tissues that actually belong in the "self" category rather than the "non-self" category. In this model, the consequences depend on where the attacked cells are and what they do. On the surface, it seems that doing anything that evokes immune system activity might make such conditions worse. Yet, transfer factors have been recommended for, and found to be effective at helping the body deal with, several putative autoimmune conditions, like rheumatoid arthritis. How might this work?

If the traditional model is correct and autoimmune conditions stem from aberrant Th2 (antibody-mediated) immune activity, transfer factors could help patients with these conditions by pulling the body back in the direction of Th1 (cell-mediated) immunity. However, it is becoming clear that many autoimmune conditions do not arise, at least not initially, from overactive Th2 responses. Rather, they involve high levels of Th1-mediated immune function, noted by high levels of the Th1 cytokine, INFγ. Understanding how and why transfer factors can be useful in such conditions requires a bit more exploration.

Marshall and Marshall (2004) suggest that high levels of INFγ in some autoimmune conditions indicate the presence of immune battles against intracellular pathogens. If this is the case, antibodies considered autoantibodies might actually be antibodies directed at remnants of self cells and pathogens left in the wake of the Th1 battle and are secondary to the underlying Th1-related inflammation. If such conditions do involve heightened but insufficient Th1 immune activity, transfer factors could be useful in treating such conditions by directly strengthening the Th1 response and helping the body rid itself of the offending intracellular pathogens. The fact that current treatments for some autoimmune conditions involve the use of synthetic INFγ supports this model, as supplemental INFγ, like transfer factors, strengthens the Th1 response.

Transfer factors might also influence autoimmune activity via mechanisms other than those leading to a strengthening of the Th1 response. Dr. Lawrence reported that Dialyzable Leukocyte Extract contains different types of transfer factors. He called one type, or fraction, *inducer factor*. These are the transfer factors that activate Th1-mediated responses aimed at fighting disease. Another type, *suppressor factor*, includes transfer factors that seem to calm down an overactive immune response, perhaps by activating Suppressor T-cells, and could be the basis for the ability of transfer factors to help some patients with some autoimmune conditions. In the words of Dr. Lawrence himself (Lawrence and Borkowsky, 1996):

> "When non-immune leucocyte populations are cultured with Inducer Factor they acquire the capacity to respond to specific antigen... When immune leucocyte populations are cultured with Suppressor Factor their response to specific antigen is blocked"

The possibility that suppressor factors might play a role in ameliorating symptoms of autoimmune conditions is strengthened by research involving laboratory animals. In 1994, Stancikova and colleagues reported that suppressor factors, which they call the *suppressor fraction* of Dialyzable Leukocyte Extract, was superior to other transfer factor fractions from

Dialyzable Leukocyte Extract at improving biological markers of arthritis in adjuvant-arthritic rats. (Adjuvant-arthritis is an experimentally induced form of arthritis in lab animals.)

It is also possible that the Th1 activation and high levels of INFγ seen in some autoimmune conditions indicate something other than intracellular infections. Steinman (2007) suggests that the recently characterized Th17 cells could be responsible for some autoimmune conditions. The Th1 response, INFγ in particular, appears to antagonize Th17 cells. As such, high levels of INFγ could be an indication that the body is attempting to reign in an aberrant Th17 response rather than indicating intracellular infections. Both synthetic INFγ and transfer factors might help some autoimmune conditions by helping the body suppress these Th17 cells. More research is needed.

Autoimmune conditions remain poorly understood. Research reviewed in Chapter 4 suggests transfer factors benefit patients with some conditions, such as rheumatoid arthritis, but not other conditions, like MS. The utility of using transfer factors for autoimmune conditions should become clearer as information accrues regarding how autoimmune conditions, and transfer factors, work.

3.8 Transfer factors, colostrinin and proline rich polypeptides – All the same?

In the early 1970s, researchers in Poland began studying the immunomodulating effects of a colostrum fraction called colostrinin. The peptides in colostrinin are called proline-rich polypeptides (PRPs), as they are rich in the amino acid, proline.

Are PRPs the same as transfer factors? Perhaps. Transfer factors are colostrum peptides weighing less than 10 kDa, and probably closer to 6 kDa (Kirkpatrick and Rozzo,

1995). PRPs are also colostrum peptides weighing less than 10 kDa (Sokolowska et al., 2007), and probably closer to 6 kDa (Kruzel et al., 2001).

Like transfer factors, PRPs appear to have powerful effects on immune activity, particularly on cells and cytokines in the Th1 response pathway. Several fascinating studies have examined the structure and function of PRPs in great detail. While research on transfer factors has focused exclusively on their roles in immune function, research on PRPs has also examined their ability to affect cognitive function and behavior. Early research suggests that PRPs are capable of improving cognitive functioning in aging animals (Popik, 2001; Stewart and Banks, 2006) and could be of benefit in Alzheimer's disease (Leszek et al., 2002; Bilikiewicz and Gaus, 2004; Stewart, 2008; Szaniszlo et al., 2009). Whether transfer factor preparations have similar effects on age-related declines in cognitive function and Alzheimer's dementia is unknown, but seems likely given the similarity between transfer factors and PRPs.

If transfer factors and PRPs are one and the same, research conducted thus far on PRPs will shed additional, important light on how these colostrum fractions work and how they could be used to improve public health.

3.8 Summary

In this chapter, we discussed what transfer factors are, how they were discovered, and how they work. Here is a summary of what we covered:

- Transfer factors are present in extracts from white blood cells and are named for their ability to transfer cell-mediated immunity from one person to another.

- They were discovered in the 1940s by NYU immunologist Dr. H. Sherwood Lawrence, MD.

- It is now known that transfer factors are small peptides and, perhaps, bits of RNA.

- Transfer factors, like antibodies, bind to antigens. While antibodies bind to antigens on pathogens floating freely in blood and lymph, transfer factors bind to antigens on the surface of infected self cells.

- Transfer factors extracted from mammalian colostrum and egg yolks appear comparable to those found in human white blood cells.

- Whether taken orally or injected, transfer factors augment the cell-mediated (Th1) immune response, as evidenced by an increase in Th1 cytokines, such as INFγ, and an increase in Th1-related immune cells, such as Natural Killer cells, Helper T-cells and Cytotoxic T-cells.

- It appears that a particular subtype of transfer factors augments the activity of Suppressor T-cells and might be of use for autoimmune conditions.

- Transfer factors are helpful in helping the body defeat existing infections and can be used to immunize the public against infectious diseases.

- Transfer factors appear to be synonymous with proline-rich polypeptides, or colostrinin, also known to have potent immunomodulating effects.

In the next chapter, we will take a close look at published research on transfer factors and explore their utility in helping the body defeat infectious diseases.

Chapter 4

Research on transfer factors in disease treatment and prevention

In the last half-century, hundreds of published studies have examined the ability of transfer factors to help the body deal with diseases. Many of them have been wildly successful while others have failed. Until recently, standardized protocols for creating highly purified, stable preparations of transfer factors did not exist, making it difficult to conduct new studies or to determine why some previous studies failed. Such standardized procedures now exist, which should facilitate future research on the utility of transfer factors in disease treatment and prevention and make it easier to evaluate the outcomes of such studies.

In the current chapter, we will explore the findings of research on transfer factors and disease. For simplicity, discussions will be organized by the reason for using transfer factor preparations — to treat diseases or prevent them. Under those categories, findings will be organized by disease type. Abstracts for all of the studies discussed in this chapter, and many more, can be found in Appendix I.

Before we begin, it is important to discuss the use of the term "treat" in this chapter and others. It is not legal to use the term when referring to supplements, as only drugs approved by the FDA can be said to treat diseases. The rule itself is in the public's best interest, though application of the rule is not always so. In the previous chapter, we discussed the mechanisms by which transfer factors affect health. They do so only by aiding the immune system and are incapable of influencing disease states without acting *through* the immune system. Thus, in this chapter, when we discuss how transfer factors are helpful in "treating" disease states, this is merely shorthand for "how transfer factors *aid the immune system* in fighting diseases."

With that caveat aside, let us examine the utility of transfer factors in disease treatment and prevention. We will begin by examining the successes and failures of transfer factors against broad, complicated disease states with poorly understood and variable etiology – including cancers, ME/CFS, multiple sclerosis and others. We will then explore the utility of transfer factors in the treatment of specific infections – including those caused by herpes viruses, fungi, mycobacteria, cell-wall deficient (CWD) bacteria and other pathogens. Finally, we will focus on one of the areas of disease management where transfer factors truly shine – the prevention of diseases via the transfer of immunity from one individual to the next.

4.1 Disease treatment

A search of MedLine/PubMed (www.pubmed.gov) for work on transfer factors yields roughly 1000 relevant publications spanning more than 50 years. Of those studies, 600 examined the therapeutic value of transfer factors in disease treatment and prevention. By all accounts, casting a wider net reveals thousands more relevant publications. We will explore studies utilizing transfer factors in disease treatment here, restricting our focus to articles indexed in MedLine/PubMed.

Cancer research

Nearly 100 studies have been conducted on the effects of transfer factors on cancer, either in patients suffering from cancer, or on cancerous cells in *in vitro* preparations – such as cancer cells grown in laboratories. Cancerous cells are those that divide aberrantly, encroaching on the space of neighboring cells, stealing their resources, and interfering with the ability of the body to function normally.

Cancerous cells are often delineated on the basis of their potential to do damage to the body, and by the type of cells involved. For instance, *leukemia* is a form of cancer caused by aberrantly dividing white blood cells (leukocytes) in the blood stream. *Lymphomas* involve aberrant division of immune cells in lymph nodes. Cancers in fat, bone or muscle cells are known as *sarcomas*. Cancers of the lung, breast, colon, bladder and prostate are known as *carcinomas*.

Cancer begins with a single cell that continues to divide when it should stop. This can happen because something triggers the cell division, or the signal that should tell the cell to die (i.e., enter apoptosis) is faulty. Hopefully, as the process of aberrant division unfolds, the proteins in the cell membrane change in ways that allow immune cells, particularly lymphocytes, to identify these "self cells" as "non-self" cells and destroy them.

Based on *in vitro* (laboratory) studies, there can be little doubt that transfer factors facilitate the ability of lymphocytes to destroy cancerous tissue. In 2006, researchers in Mexico examined the ability of Dialyzable Leukocyte Extract taken from white blood cells from cows to prevent breast cancer cells from further division and to facilitate their destruction (Franco-Molina et al, 2006). The experiment was successful, and the researchers demonstrated a dose-dependent effect of the Dialyzable Leuko-cyte Extract on cancer cells, meaning that more Dialyzable Leukocyte Extract led to greater destruction of cancer cells. The Dialyzable Leukocyte Extract had no impact on normal, healthy cells, only cancerous cells, indicating that the constituents of the extract, transfer factors, specifically help the immune system deal with pathogens and do not damage healthy tissue. Dozens of other *in vitro* studies examining the effects of transfer factor-containing extracts on cancer cells have demonstrated similar results, as have studies done *in vivo* – that is, in living animals, including humans.

In 2005, Pineda and colleagues (Pineda et al, 2005) re-ported on a fascinating study in which they examined the impact of transfer factors on glioma — brain cancer involving glial cells — in rats. Here is what they found:

> "TF reduced significantly the tumour size, and increased CD2+, CD4+, CD8+ and NK cell counts, it also increased the percentage of apop-totic [dying] tumour cells"

While rats are not humans, these data are extremely promising. Smaller tumors and increased levels of four types of lymphocytes involved in cell-mediated immunity!

Dozens of studies have examined the ability of transfer factors to help humans suffering from cancers of various types. In 1996, the Italian researcher Giancarlo Pizza and his colleagues (Pizza et al, 1996) reported on efforts to treat a form of prostate cancer typically unresponsive to conventional therapies. The authors generated transfer factors that bind to antigens on prostate cancer cells and injected them into sick patients once each month. In the words of the authors,

> "As conventional treatments are unsuccessful, the survival rate of stage D3 prostate cancer pa-

tients is poor. Reports have suggested the existence of humoral and cell-mediated immunity
(CMI) against prostate cancer tumour-associated
antigens (TAA). These observations prompted us
to treat stage D3 prostate cancer patients with an
in vitro produced transfer factor (TF) able to
transfer, in vitro and in vivo, CMI against bladder
and prostate TAA. Fifty patients entered this
study and received one intramuscular injection of
2-5 units of specific TF monthly. Follow-up,
ranging from 1 to 9 years, showed that complete
remission was achieved in 2 patients, partial remission in 6, and no progression of metastatic
disease in 14. The median survival was 126
weeks, higher than the survival rates reported in
the literature for patients of the same stage."

Thus, compared to the expected length of survival for
men with this form of prostate cancer, it appears that transfer
factor treatment significantly prolonged the life of patients in the
study. Though such findings are promising, the lack of a true
control group – a group receiving everything else but the transfer
factors – makes it difficult to determine the role that transfer
factors actually played in the patients' disease progression.

During that same year, Pizza and colleagues (Pilotti et al,
1996) reported on a study in which a control group was used.
Ninety-nine patients with small cell lung cancer were given
transfer factors and their survival times were compared to 257
patients with lung cancer who were not given transfer factors.
Those given transfer factors survived significantly longer than
those not given the treatment.

Wagner and colleagues (Wagner et al, 1987) reported on
a study in which 32 female patients with cervical cancer were
treated with transfer factors derived from their husband's white
blood cells while 28 patients with cervical cancer were not.

Within a two year period following hysterectomy to remove the cancerous tissue, cancer returned in 40% (11/28) of subjects in the control group compared to only 15% (5/32) of subjects in the transfer factor group.

When taken as a whole, studies on the effectiveness of transfer factors against cancer strongly suggest that they help destroy cancer cells in the laboratory and can be effective for some patients under some circumstances in real life. However, it is important to point out exactly how variable the outcomes of research on this topic have been. Indeed, during the same year that the above study was published, Spitler and Miller (1987) published a critical review of the literature on transfer factor therapy for cancer. Here is what they concluded:

> "Results of clinical trials of transfer factor therapy in various malignancies have been variable. In non randomized trials, about 300 patients have been evaluated, and clinical benefit has been reported in about 1/3 of the evaluable patients. Results of randomized studies are similarly varied. In some randomized trials, clinical benefits of increased disease free survival and prolonged survival have been claimed. In other studies, transfer factor has been reported to be of no clinical benefit… This review of the literature regarding the clinical effort of transfer factor in malignancy leads to the conclusion that transfer factor might not be an effective therapy of cancer. If it does have efficacy in certain malignancies, it is unlikely that it will alone have dramatic effects in substantial numbers of patients. Perhaps transfer factor may have a role in tumor therapy as an adjuvant to other forms of therapy and as surgery, irradiation, or chemotherapy. In order for the proper evaluation of transfer factor in reproducible

comparative studies, it will be necessary to have a standardized reproducible product which can be assessed by appropriate quality control procedures."

As alluded to in the last sentence, the studies on which the article is based were written prior to the development of standardized protocols for obtaining highly purified and potent transfer factor extracts. Such techniques were developed in the 1990s. Hopefully, now that such preparations are available, large scale studies of the utility of transfer factors in cancer treatment eventually will be funded and conducted. At the very least, studies performed in the last decade or so seem to hold promise that such an approach could prolong the lives of cancer patients, if not reversing the progression of the disease.

During cancer treatment with radiation and chemotherapy, healthy body cells pay a massive toll, particularly those that replicate quickly. Indeed, it is partly because these treatments tend to affect cells during division that they can be effective at killing the cancer before killing the host. In order to wage a war against pathogens, immune cells must divide quickly. As such, radiation and chemotherapy can severely weaken the ability of the immune system to do its job.

Because transfer factors are able to stimulate the creation of new lymphocytes, it makes sense that they might be effective at helping to repair the damage done to the immune system by cancer treatment. That is exactly what researchers in Cuba observed. Fernandez and colleagues (Fernandez et al, 1993) examined the impact of transfer factors on immune markers in eight patients undergoing chemotherapy for leukemia. Measurements from these patients were compared to those from 14 control patients undergoing chemotherapy for leukemia but not receiving transfer factors. Transfer factors sped the recovery of numbers of white blood cells and the incidence of opportunistic infections during treatment was lower in the transfer factor group relative to controls.

In 2004, researchers from the Russian Ministry of Health reported on the benefits of using commercially available transfer factor preparations to aid recovery in patients following surgery for gastric cancer. Levels of important immune cells and cytokines were raised and lowered in ways suggesting a strengthening and rebalancing of immune activity. According to the report:

> "Twenty-five (25) patients (the treatment or main group) with second or third clinical stage of gastric cancer participated in clinical studies of TF PLUS... Twenty-five (25) patients of sex, age, nosology, and matched disease stage comprised the control group. All of the gastric cancer patients in both groups underwent surgical treatment and during the postoperative period the standard procedure of immunotherapeutic treatment. To stimulate non-specific immunity, patients in the treatment group received TF PLUS, 1 capsule 3 times daily for 30 days, along with the standard treatment... After the end of the course of complex treatment the study was continued with TF PLUS administration and it demonstrated that the continued treatment was beneficial to immune, interferon and cytokine status, as well as for the clinical improvement of the patients. There was an increase of CD3+, CD4+ and CD8+ content in blood lymphocyte populations and the number of NK cells in blood samples markedly increased both showing activation of the cell mediated immunity. Concerning humoral immunity, positive changes towards normal levels of TNF-a and IL-1b production were registered."

In another recent study, Franco-Melina et al. (2008) provide additional, compelling evidence that transfer factors are powerful adjuvants in the treatment of cancer. Twenty-four patients with non-small cell lung cancer (NSCLC) were divided into two groups – one receiving standard chemotherapy for cancer and the other receiving standard therapy plus a transfer factor preparation called ImmunePotent CRP. Transfer factors had a clear impact on the outcome. In the words of the authors,

> "The administration of IMMUNEPOTENT CRP induced immunomodulatory activity (increasing the total leukocytes and T-lymphocyte subpopulations CD4(+), CD8(+), CD16(+) and CD56(+), and maintaining DHT) and increased the quality of the patients' lives, suggesting immunologic protection against chemotherapeutic side-effects in NSCLC patients... Our results suggest the possibility of using IMMUNEPOTENT CRP alongside radiation and chemotherapy for maintaining the immune system and increasing the quality of life of the patients."

Additional research indicates that transfer factors could play an important role in helping cancer patients beat opportunistic infections that arise as a result of suppressed immune function. According to the authors (Ketchel et al, 1979):

> "We used transfer factor in the treatment of 15 patients, most with leukemia, who had fungal, viral, or mycobacterial infections that were not responding to conventional therapy. Seven of ten evaluable patients had therapeutic control of their infections while receiving transfer factor. Transfer factor appears to have contributed to

these clinical improvements and is a modality of treatment that deserves further investigation."

Thus, in addition to their potential effectiveness as adjunct treatments for cancer, transfer factors help protect cancer patients from infections during chemotherapy, as well as helping the immune system heal itself from the damage that surgery and chemotherapy can do.

Myalgic Encephalomyelitis/Chronic Fatigue Syndrome

Myalgic Encephalomyelitis/Chronic Fatigue Syndrome (ME/CFS) is a condition known by many names, including Chronic Fatigue Immune Dysfunction Syndrome (CFIDS) and Chronic Fatigue Syndrome (CFS). The condition is characterized by intermittent cognitive impairments (brain fog), widespread physical discomfort, dizziness upon standing, aching fatigue, poor sleep and other symptoms. Its etiology is unknown, and can either develop slowly over time or begin abruptly, often following a viral illness.

> The combination of **myalgic** and **encephalomyelitis** means "painful inflammation in the brain and spinal cord"

In many cases, it appears that ME/CFS sufferers exhibit insufficient Th1 (cell-mediated) immune system activity, perhaps combined with chronic activation of some aspects of the Th2 (antibody-mediated) immune response. Recall that the Th1 immune response involves activation of macrophages, Cytotoxic T-cells and Natural Killer cells in order to attack cells infected with viruses and bacteria. A recent report by Dr. Nancy Klimas, considered an authority on ME/CFS, suggests that female ME/CFS sufferers can be sorted according to Natural Killer cell levels. Those with below normal levels tend to exhibit greater levels of cognitive dysfunction, reduced drive, and greater difficulties functioning during the day.

Inherent or acquired weaknesses in the Th1 branch of the immune response would place patients at risk of becoming infested with opportunistic pathogens. A large percentage of ME/CFS patients test positive for active infections with HHV-6, one of eight strains of herpes viruses, as well as the recently identified retrovirus, XMRV (Fan, 2007; Lombardi et al., 2009).

The link between HHV-6 infections and at least some symptoms of ME/CFS is strengthened by evidence that valganciclovir, a form the antiviral acyclovir, seems to improve the symptoms of ME/CFS in some patients infected with HHV-6 (Kogelnik et al, 2006). In a subsequent section, we will discuss evidence that recurring intense headaches and diffuse back pain can be brought on by infections in the spinal and cranial nerves by several different variants of herpes viruses, including HHV-6. It is possible this could explain some of the myalgia associated with ME/CFS. We will return to this topic shortly.

One of the most frustrating aspects of ME/CFS for those who suffer from it is something called *post-exertional malaise*. Despite their desire to exercise and strengthen their bodies, many patients with this condition cannot. For them, exercise often exacerbates the problems rather than promoting health. The CDC defines the phenomenon of post-exertional malaise as a "relapse of symptoms after physical or mental exertion". This effectively traps the sick individual and confines them to light duties, if those are possible.

Research indicates that Th1-related immune system markers, such as the number of Natural Killer cells, increase following exercise of moderate intensity. As mentioned above, many patients with ME/CFS show low Natural Killer cell levels at baseline. Perhaps exercise temporarily strengthens the Th1-mediated immune response, allowing the immune system to ratchet up its efforts to rid the individual of whatever pathogens have set up shop. This could lead to an increase in sick behaviors and the experiences that go with it as the intensity of the battle increases. Because the body still cannot overcome the pathogens, the individual simply feels sicker for a day or two – what the CDC refers to as a relapse in this case – before eventually returning to their normal, sick state.

Given the ability of transfer factors to increase levels of Cytotoxic T-cells, macrophages and Natural Killer cells, it seems logical to postulate that ME/CFS sufferers, particularly those with low Natural Killer cell counts, would benefit greatly from transfer factor therapy. Enhancing the Th1-mediated immune response could have a normalizing effect on immune function by reducing the magnitude of Th2 activity and the symptoms that result (allergies, some autoimmune activity, etc). The value of normalizing Th1/Th2 responses in ME/CFS sufferers is discussed by Nancy Klimas and colleagues in a 2001 review of treatment strategies for the disorder, referred to by the more basic title of Chronic Fatigue Syndrome or CFS (Patarca-Monero et al, 2001):

> "Patients with CFS who show evidence of activation of the immune system have poor immune cell function and a predominance of what is called a T-helper (Th)2-type cytokine response when their lymphocytes are activated. A Th2-type response, which is characterized by production of cytokines such as interleukin (IL)-4, -5, and -10, favours the function of B lymphocytes, the cellular factories of immunoglobulins. A predominance of a Th2-type response is therefore consistent with pathologies, such as autoimmunity and atopy, which are based on inappropriate production of immunoglobulins. Many of the CFS therapies discussed decrease the Th2-type predominance seen at baseline in CFS patients, thereby allowing a greater predominance of a Th1-type response, which favours the function of macrophages and natural killer cells. The function of the latter cells, which have the natural ability of directly destroying invading microbes

and cancer cells, is defective in untreated CFS patients."

Some well-known treatments for ME/CFS, including Ampligen, Kutapressin, and Isoprinosine (Imunovir) all seem to have the ability to shift the balance of immune responses from Th2 > Th1 back toward a balance of Th2 and Th1. Researchers at the University of Aberdeen in Scotland (Williams et al, 2005) recently reported that antibiotic therapy, which seems to improve general well-being in some ME/CFS patients, either amplifies both Th1 and Th2 cytokine expression, as is the case with moxifloxacin and ciprofloxacin, or amplifies predominantly Th1-related cytokine expression, as is the case with clarithromycin. Both of these effects might help normalize the Th1/Th2 profile. It is also possible the improvements brought on by antibiotics reflect the existence of underlying bacterial infections.

The substances discussed above – including Ampligen, Kutapressin and Isoprinosine – influence the Th1/Th2 ratio indirectly and are insufficient for many patients. Transfer factors, on the other hand, are powerful Th1 stimulators that do so directly using a language that immune cells inherently understand.

Despite the logic of using transfer factors in ME/CFS therapy, relatively few studies have been done on the topic to date, and the underlying immune conditions in subjects in those studies were not well-characterized, making it difficult to determine reasons for success and failure in individual patients. Regardless, the existing, though limited, science strongly suggests that transfer factors could work quite well for some ME/CFS patients. It seems likely that future studies conducted with newly available standardized transfer factors, including those that target HHV-6 and other viruses common in this condition, will yield more consistent results.

In 1996, Paul Levine from the National Cancer Institute in Bethesda, Maryland, published three studies on the use of transfer factors in the treatment of ME/CFS. All of the articles appeared in a single issue of the journal, *Biotherapy*. Two of the papers were co-authored by Italian researcher Giancarlo Pizza and his colleagues. Only one other study, in addition to the three by Levine, has explored the possibility of using transfer factors in the treatment of ME/CFS.

In the first of the three papers by Dr. Levine, he suggests that transfer factors specific to herpes viruses — including Epstein-Barr virus (EBV), human herpes virus-6 (HHV-6), and cytomegalovirus (CMV) — could be beneficial for ME/CFS sufferers given the tendency for many such patients to test positive for these pathogens. The other two manuscripts report on small studies in which the researchers treated ME/CFS sufferers with transfer factor therapy.

In one of the studies, Ablashi and colleagues (1996) treated two patients who tested positive for HHV-6 with transfer factors with specificity for the virus. The first patient was a 24-year-old male student. Along with the HHV-6 infection, the patient tested positive for elevated CMV antibodies and experienced typical symptoms associated with ME/CFS. Interestingly, in this patient, levels of Natural Killer cells were elevated, rather than suppressed as is often reported in ME/CFS patients.

The second patient was a 27-year-old female student who presented with symptoms of ME/CFS, including headaches, difficulty concentrating, memory problems, and depression. Her symptoms also included sore throat and tender lymph nodes, symptoms not always present in ME/CFS patients. She tested positive for an active HHV-6 infection, as well as an EBV infection

In patient one, test results suggested that the HHV-6 infection subsided after two months of treatment with transfer factors. Similarly, in patient two, both the HHV-6 and EBV infections cleared up over the course of five months of treatment.

Clinically, patient one did not show any signs of improvement, despite resolution of the HHV-6 infection. In contrast, patient two showed dramatic improvements in health. In the words of the study authors:

"The second patient continued to improve physically and eventually she resumed normal activities. Her condition, two years later, is absolutely normal."

The reason why patient two, but not patient one, improved is unknown. However, differences in clinical markers of improvement between the two patients should not be surprising, as the clinical symptoms they exhibited at the study onset were quite different. They shared some clinical symptoms (e.g., fatigue) but not others (e.g., patient two had a sore throat and swollen lymph nodes but patient one did not). Both had active infections with HHV-6, but only patient two tested positive for EBV. Who knows what else differed between the two patients.

In a second study by Levine and colleagues (De Vinci et al, 1996), transfer factors were given to 20 patients with ME/CFS. Twelve patients received transfer factors with known specificity against CMV and EBV (TF prep 1), six received broad spectrum transfer factors (TF prep 2), one patient received transfer factors with specificity against EBV and HHV-6 (TF prep 3), and one received TF prep 1 and then TF prep 3. It appears that some subjects, perhaps all, were administered transfer factor preparations in oral form.

Unfortunately, while the authors indicate that the study involved a "placebo controlled design", it clearly did not. All patients received transfer factors. Just the time course of treatment and the nature of the transfer factor extracts used differed between patients.

Seven of 12 patients receiving TF prep 1 exhibited clinical improvements, as did 3 of 6 receiving TF prep 2, and both patients administered TF prep 3 (including the subject who was given TF prep 1 and then TF prep 3). These improvements included diminished sore throat, diminished muscle and/or joint pain, diminished headaches, and improved mental concentration. While not listed, it is presumed that the level of fatigue was also a variable of interest given the patients' diagnoses. One patient dropped out due to apparent worsening of symptoms, while one dropped out due to developing acne, despite marked improvements in the clinical picture. As in the previous study, clinical improvement did not necessarily correspond with changes in the presence of HHV-6, CMV or EBV.

Overall, despite the fact that the study was imperfect from a methodological standpoint, and that subjects presented with diverse clinical symptoms and viral infections, transfer factors appeared to be of great benefit for more than half (60%) of the subjects.

In the third and final study involving the use of transfer factors to treat patients with symptoms consistent with ME/CFS, researchers in Prague (Hana et al., 1996) assessed the impact of transfer factors on 222 patients suffering from Cellular Immunodeficiency (CID), some with debilitating fatigue and or EBV and CMV infections. Essentially, CID is any condition that involves deficient immune system function. It could involve suppressed Th1 (cell-mediated) and/or suppressed Th2 (antibody-mediated) immune activity.

Subjects were given a total of 6 injections of transfer factors over the course of 8 weeks. Measures of immune system function were taken before and after this 8-week period. For those with viral infections, immunoglobulin-G was added, as well as vitamin supplements.

Subjects in the study ranged in age from 17-77, a broad range. To tease out the influence of age on treatment effectiveness, the researchers divided subjects, and their data, into three groups — 17 to 43 (123 subjects), 44 to 53 (52 subjects), and 54 to 77 (47 subjects).

Transfer factor therapy was very effective in a large percentage of patients, both in terms of reduced viral activity, increased T-cell counts, and improvements in clinical symptoms. Interestingly, there were clear differences in the effectiveness of transfer factors depending on age group. In the words of the authors (words in brackets were added for clarification):

> "Examination of clinical status of patients after Immodin [transfer factor] therapy show the following results: in group A [youngest group], 98/123 patients were in complete recovery and 12 partially improved, whilst 13/123 (10.6%) did not. In group B [middle age range group], 27/52 recovered completely, 19 partially and 6 (11.5%) showed no improvement. In group C [oldest group], 15 patients recovered completely, 18 partially, and 14 patients (29.8%) failed to improve."

Data from the study clearly suggest that transfer factors helped subjects, particularly younger subjects, recover. Indeed, the majority of young patients were considered to be "cured" by the researchers, meaning that all clinical symptoms (e.g., fatigue, headaches, muscle pain, etc) went away. This is very promising, particularly for younger patients.

With regard to the increase in T-cell counts following transfer factor therapy, the pattern was consistent with the pattern of age-related clinical improvements. Clinical improvements were seen in 89, 88, and 70% of subjects from youngest to oldest. Increased T-cell counts were observed in 89, 79, and 40% of subjects from youngest to oldest. Such age-related effects could stem from the fact that T-cell counts, and immune system health in general, decrease as we get older. Perhaps the immune system in older subjects is simply less responsive to immunomodulators like transfer factors.

The condition studied in the above experiment, CID, is not the same as ME/CFS, but probably captures a particular subset of ME/CFS sufferers – those with low lymphocyte counts. As mentioned previously, it seems that some ME/CFS patients exhibit low lymphocyte counts while others do not. Data from the study on CID patients, along with data from the two smaller studies discussed before it, provide compelling reasons to expect that transfer factors might be particularly beneficial to those ME/CFS sufferers with low lymphocyte – including T-cell and Natural Killer cell – counts.

Currently, there are no accepted laboratory markers for ME/CFS. However, for those who suffer from the condition, a test for levels of Natural Killer cells could help them make an informed decision regarding whether to include transfer factors in their treatment regimen. Again, based on the available, but limited, data, it seems that those with low counts might be particularly good candidates for benefiting from the immune boosting properties of transfer factors.

Additional research on the utility of transfer factors in treating ME/CFS seems warranted. It is now clear that there are links between ME/CFS, herpes infections, and weakened Th1-mediated immunity. It is also clear that transfer factors have tremendous utility in treating herpes viruses (data reviewed in a subsequent section) and strengthening Th1-mediated immune responses. Collectively, these are compelling reasons to fund and conduct well-controlled studies on the efficacy of transfer factors for treating subsets of ME/CFS patients with active herpes infections and/or weakened Th1 immunity.

As discussed in the last chapter, scientific dogma is slow to change. In 2006, the CDC launched a campaign to educate the public about ME/CFS, which they still call Chronic Fatigue Syndrome (CFS), and to assess the underlying basis of the condition. It is too early to determine how much fruit the initiative will yield.

Fibromyalgia

ME/CFS and fibromyalgia (FM) are often mentioned in the same breath. While these conditions share many overlapping symptoms — including fatigue, headaches, brain-fog, irritable bowel syndrome, sleep disturbances and others — there are several features that set the conditions apart. Most of these differences have to do with chronic, heightened pain sensitivity throughout the body, and tenderness in specific body areas, for those suffering from FM. There are 18 points on the body (9 on each side) that tend to be extremely tender in patients with FM. These points are spaced between the back of the head behind the ear down to the insides of the knees. The guidelines offered by the American College of Rheumatology require that a patient exhibit tenderness in 11 or more points in order to be diagnosed with FM.

To date, no studies have been conducted examining the utility of transfer factors for FM, though there must have been some FM patients mixed in with subjects in other studies. While recent research on ME/CFS has focused on immune system dysfunction, work on FM has honed in on underlying problems with pain signal processing in the brain and spinal cord, as well as pain generation in the muscles themselves. Neurons (a type of brain cell) involved in the transmission of pain signals appear to become sensitized to pain signals in FM patients, meaning that these cells are very responsive to pain signals, perhaps effectively amplifying them. There also appear to be differences between healthy control subjects and FM patients with regard to patterns of dopamine (a chemical messenger used by brain cells) released in the brain. Dopamine exerts its effects on brain activity by plugging into specialized receptors on neurons. The ultimate role that dopamine plays in behavior and experience depends on where, in the brain, the dopamine is acting. Dopamine levels in some areas are associated with feeling pleasure, in others dopamine is involved in movement, and in others it influences the perception of pain.

Researchers from the McGill University Centre for Research on Pain (Woode et al, 2007) recently reported that patients with FM show a blunted dopamine increase in specific brain areas, including the basal ganglia, in response to pain. In healthy controls, higher levels of reported pain were associated with higher levels of dopamine release. Not so in patients with FM. Indeed, they reported higher levels of pain than controls but released less dopamine in the basal ganglia. Some FM patients showed little or no detectable change in dopamine levels.

Reduced dopamine release in the basal ganglia could help explain another recent finding from a different laboratory. Researchers in Germany (Schmidt-Wilcke et al, 2007) reported finding increases in gray matter volumes in the basal ganglia of patients with FM. Gray matter reflects parts of neurons, the cells that receive dopamine signals. If dopamine levels are low in the basal ganglia, neurons waiting for dopamine signals would be expected to branch out, effectively becoming larger, in an effort to pick up the weak dopamine signals. Theoretically, this would lead to an increase in gray matter there. Thus, if patients with FM have limited dopamine levels in the basal ganglia, an increase in gray matter volumes might be expected.

The link between low dopamine levels and heightened pain in patients with FM could also help explain the effectiveness of some antidepressants at reducing pain for many FM sufferers. The effect is traditionally interpreted as stemming from increased serotonin levels. This might be true given the involvement of serotonin in regulating pain signal processing in the spinal cord. However, the effects might also stem from increases in dopamine levels in the brain. All antidepressants appear to increase levels of dopamine, including those labeled as Selective Serotonin Reuptake Inhibitors (SSRIs).

If low dopamine levels really do play a role in the pain experienced by FM sufferers, then raising dopamine levels should dampen the pain. In 2005, Washington D.C. rheumatologists Holman and Myers reported that 42% of FM sufferers who received pramipexole, a drug that increases dopamine levels in the brain, experienced >50% reduction in pain levels over a 14 week period. In contrast, only 14% of those receiving placebo exhibited similar reductions in pain (Holman and Myers, 2005).

Many patients with FM are currently being treated with drugs like Wellbutrin (bupropion), an antidepressant, or Provigil (modafinil), an anti-narcolepsy drug, for their fatigue. Both drugs primarily act by increasing dopamine levels (Murillo-Rodriguez et al, 2007). It would be of interest to determine whether such patients also receive relief from pain.

Clearly, research into the mechanisms underlying ME/CFS and FM are heading in different directions. Recent studies suggest that, at one level, the pathology underlying FM might rest in the processing of pain signals in the brain and spinal cord, perhaps involving diminished dopamine release and changes in the size and structure of certain brain areas. It is possible that the pathology underlying FM, like that of many cases of ME/CFS, results from infection or immune dysfunction, but this remains to be determined.

Given the safety profile of supplemental transfer factors and the potential that they might be of benefit, taking them for a few months under a doctor's supervision is the best way to determine if they would be helpful in individual cases of FM.

Rheumatoid arthritis

Rheumatoid arthritis (RA) is one of 100 or so conditions that fall under the general canopy of arthritis – which means "joint inflammation." The causes of arthritis are as varied as the conditions bearing its name.

RA is a chronic, debilitating condition in which the body appears to attack self cells in the joints, causing inflammation and pain. Somewhere between 50-95% of adult RA sufferers test positive for heightened levels of "rheumatoid factor", or IgM RF. You might recall from the first chapter that immunoglobulin is another term for antibody. The presence of high levels of

IgM RF suggests, at least to some researchers, that the inflammation is caused by an elevated and aberrant Th2 (antibody-mediated) response in which antibodies direct immune cells to attack "self-cells".

The ends of bones in each moveable joint in the body are covered with a membrane called the synovium. Rheumatoid arthritis is thought to occur when immune cells enter the fluid under the synovium, attack self cells and cause inflammation. Other researchers believe the inflammation is triggered by a Th1 response aimed at intracellular pathogens in the inflamed area rather than by a Th2-driven generation of autoantibodies.

One of the pro-inflammatory cytokines involved in the immune response associated with RA is the Th1 cytokine, *tumor necrosis factor*, or TNF. Many current approaches offered by drug companies for managing RA focus on reducing levels of TNF. These drugs include Enbrel, Remicade and Humira. Rather than aiming at the underlying causes of the immune activation associated with RA, these drugs act by simply suppressing the chronically activated immune system. They work wonders for treating symptoms, but it is becoming clear that the immune system suppression caused by these drugs can produce harmful side effects.

In 2006, an analysis of data from several clinical trials involving the use of Remicade and Humira (Enbrel was excluded, but is a similar drug) was published in the *Journal of the American Medical Association* by researchers at the Mayo Clinic. The analyses revealed that RA patients treated with Remicade and Humira were 3.3 times as likely to get cancer and twice as likely to get serious infections.

Such concerns are known to the manufacturers of TNF blocking drugs, as well as the FDA. This is made clear in information, included on the following page, from the Enbrel website (www.enbrel.com). Side effects are said to include, "serious nervous system disorders, such as multiple sclerosis, seizures, or inflammation of the nerves of the eyes." Also, please note the mis-use of the word *treat* in the text box about Enbrel. It is hardly the case that immunosuppressants *treat* diseases, rather they help manage symptoms. That is, no one has ever been cured of a disease by an immunosuppressant. Indeed, if the position of Marshall and Marshall (2004) is correct and many putative autoimmune conditions are actually caused by an aggravated but insufficient Th1 response aimed at intracellular pathogens, suppressing the Th1 response with TNF blocking agents would only prolong and perhaps worsen the ailment.

What important information do I need to know about taking ENBREL?

ENBREL is a type of protein called a tumor necrosis factor (TNF) blocker that blocks the action of a substance your body's immune system makes called TNF. People with an immune disease, such as rheumatoid arthritis, ankylosing spondylitis, psoriatic arthritis, and psoriasis, have too much TNF in their bodies. ENBREL can reduce the amount of TNF in the body to normal levels, helping to treat your disease. But, in doing so, ENBREL can also lower the ability of your immune system to fight infections.

All medicines have side effects, including ENBREL. Possible side effects of ENBREL include...

Serious nervous system disorders, such as multiple sclerosis, seizures, or inflammation of the nerves of the eyes...

Rare reports of serious blood disorders (some fatal)...

In medical studies of all TNF blockers, including ENBREL, a higher rate of lymphoma (a type of cancer) was seen compared to the general population. The risk of lymphoma may be up to several-fold higher in rheumatoid arthritis and psoriasis patients

The role of TNF blockers, including ENBREL, in the development of lymphoma is unknown...

In a medical study of patients with JRA, infections, headaches, abdominal pain, vomiting, and nausea occurred more frequently than in adults

---

Regardless of the mechanisms underlying RA, research suggests that transfer factors are of benefit in some cases. In 1985, Georgescu reported on what remains the largest study examining the utility of transfer factors in the management of RA. Fifty female patients were followed for two years and assessed every three months. Patients were treated with non-steroidal anti-inflammatory drugs on an as-needed basis, and were injected with transfer factors once per week for the first 6 months and then once per month thereafter. The author reports that "excellent, very good and good results were obtained in 35 patients (70%)", leading him to concluded that,

> "The study confirmed the fact that specific im-
> munotherapy with TF represents an important
> adjuvant in the treatment of rheumatoid arthri-
> tis (RA)."

Three small studies, all performed in the 1970s, ex-amined the impact of transfer factors in juvenile RA — two with positive results (Kass et al, 1974; Grohn et al, 1976) and one with negative results (Hoyeraal et al, 1978). Interestingly, in the study with negative results, the transfer factor preparation used not only failed to improve the symptoms of juvenile RA, it failed to produce changes in immune activity that would be expected following transfer factor administration in general. Indeed, many of the subjects exhibited a decrease in T-cell levels, the opposite of what others consistently report with transfer factor therapy. Such findings raise questions about the viability of the transfer factor preparation used in the study.

How, exactly, transfer factors exert positive effects against RA — for those in which they do so — is unknown. As mentioned previously, they could help such conditions by pulling immune activity away from the Th2 response toward the Th1 response, thus effectively calming the autoimmune activity thought to underlie some forms of arthritis. It is also possible that transfer factors directly suppress an overactive immune response. This issue will be discussed later in the chapter. Further, it has long been speculated that some forms of arthritis are caused by infections with bacteria, which require a strong Th1 response to defeat. In such cases, transfer factors could be beneficial against arthritis by helping the body eradicate the underlying infection.

Research also suggests that transfer factors, like the pharmaceutical drugs discussed above, could reduce levels of TNF. In 2005, scientists in Cuba reported on a study in which they assessed the effects of transfer factors on levels of cyto-kines, including TNF, released by white blood cells spurred into action by lipopolysaccharide, a portion of the cell wall of bacteria (Fernandez-Ortega et al, 2005). In the presence of transfer factors from Dialyzable Leukocyte Extract, TNF release was suppressed. A similar finding was published by this same labora-tory a year earlier. The mechanisms by which this effect occurs is unclear and is counterintuitive given that transfer factors aug-ment Th1 activity and TNF is a Th1-related cytokine.

Recall that the purpose of potentially dangerous drugs like Humira, Remicade and Enbrel is to suppress TNF. Whether transfer factors are more or less effective than Humira, Remi-cade and Enbrel remains to be determined. However, given the vastly different safety profiles of these categories of substances, and the added benefits of transfer factors for immune health, transfer factors would certainly be preferable, even if their potency was less than that of the pharmaceuticals.

Multiple sclerosis – Proof that not everything can be fixed by strengthening the Th1 immune response

Multiple sclerosis (MS) is a perplexing disease. It tends to begin during adulthood but can begin during childhood or adolescence, strikes women with greater frequency than men, and occurs more often in Caucasians. If one identical twin has it, the odds are somewhere between 20-50% that the other will develop it, suggesting a genetic predisposition. As discussed in Chapter 2, Vitamin D deficiency has been implicated in MS. Indeed, in cases where one identical twin has MS, the healthy twin tends to spend more time in the sun, which is critical for Vitamin D synthesis.

The onset of MS can be slow or sudden. It is progressive, meaning that it usually worsens over time. Initially, symptoms tend to follow a pattern of relapse and remission, in which flare-ups are followed by quiescent periods. As time goes by, most patients begin to experience symptoms on a more regular, ongoing basis. The disease itself is eventually fatal in an estimated 50% of all cases, with suicide claiming the life of an additional 15% of MS sufferers.

MS is a condition in which a fatty substance called myelin, which surrounds most neurons in the brain and spinal cord, begins to disappear. Neurons communicate with each other – as well as with the muscles that move us around and allow us to speak – by releasing chemicals onto each other. The release of these chemicals begins with a tiny electrical jolt that travels down a long extension of the neuron, called an axon. The axon is like an arm reaching out to other neurons or muscles. Axons are surrounded by myelin, which is created by a major category of cells in the brain and spinal cord, the glial cells. For some reason, in MS, the myelin sheath degrades, thus demyelinating the neurons. Without the myelin, the electrical jolt cannot travel effectively down the axon. Without the electrical jolt, chemicals aren't released from one cell to the next. If the chemicals are not released, signals are not sent, and the systems affected do not work.

It is this process – poor signal transmission due to demyelination – that leads to the symptoms of MS. What those symptoms are will depend on which neurons are being demyelinated. Because problems with movement are the most obvious, MS is usually characterized as a condition that involves problems with movement. However, there can also be a litany of "hidden" symptoms, including problems with thought and emotion, depending on which areas are hit. Sexual dysfunction, including erectile dysfunction in men, and changes in sensory input from the skin, like numbness and tingling, are also common.

What causes the demyelination underlying the condition is unknown, but the common view is that it involves an autoimmune process in which the body's immune cells aberrantly attack the glial cells that form the myelin. It is also possible that these glial cells become infected and that the immune system attacks the glial cells in an effort to get rid of the infection. Antibodies considered autoantibodies could be antibodies generated against fragments of self cells and pathogens left behind after the Th1 battles against the intracellular pathogens. As with other conditions, the autoimmune label could reflect our current lack of knowledge of pathogens and the immune responses they evoke. Regardless, the diminished myelination that results is a real problem for those with MS.

It has been suggested that MS might stem from an underlying imbalance in Th1/Th2 response profiles. Because most immune conditions, no matter what their specific cause, manifest imbalances in Th1/Th2 responses as the body attempts to protect and repair itself, such characterizations are often more descriptive than explanatory. In the case of MS, immune activity seems to be tilted toward Th1 rather than Th2 as in other autoimmune conditions.

If MS is related to a general weakness or imbalance in immune function, or to an underlying intracellular infection, treating MS sufferers with substances capable of helping the body strengthen immune activity and re-establish a balance in Th1/Th2 responses, like transfer factors, might be expected to improve their prognosis. Unfortunately, this has not been the case to date. Several studies have attempted to improve the symptoms of MS via the administration of transfer factors. Failures to do so have been reported as far back as 1976. According to one report (Behan et al, 1976):

"The effect of transfer factor prepared from relatives of patients with multiple sclerosis (M.S.) and from unrelated donors on the clinical course of M.S. has been studied in fifteen male and fifteen female patients. Some patients were given transfer factor and some placebo (physiological saline). Results of three independent clinical examinations by different neurologists and subjective assessments by the patients showed no difference between those given transfer factor and those given placebo."

In 1978, the results of a more formal study in which 56 patients with MS were treated with either transfer factors or placebo in a double-blind design – meaning that no one was aware of who got what until the end of the study – for one year were reported. No improvements were observed.

It is possible that the beneficial effects of transfer factors take months, if not years, to reveal themselves. It is also possible that the general immune boosting properties of transfer factors could help slow the progression of the disease, despite its failure to reverse the clinical course of the illness. Indeed, there are several studies suggesting that this might be the case.

The results of a large, double-blind study conducted in the UK on the effectiveness of transfer factors against MS were published in 1986. The authors (Frith et al, 1986) concluded that transfer factors slowed the rate of progression of the disease, but that beneficial effects were not evident until at least 18 months after the onset of treatment. In essence, transfer factor therapy did not improve the health of MS sufferers initially, but those treated with transfer factors seemed to exhibit slightly less progression of disease severity than other MS patients.

Currently, several drugs based on natural cytokines released during inflammatory immune responses are approved by the FDA for the treatment of MS. One of them, Rebif, has been widely used for many years. Rebif, INF beta-1a, is a synthetic form of interferon, one of the many cytokines used by Th1-related immune cells to communicate. Interferon is released by immune cells in response to viral or bacterial infections. It stimulates the production of Cytotoxic T-cells, Natural Killer cells and macrophages, pulling the body toward more Th1 activity. Interferon essentially informs new and existing immune cells that a pathogen is present. Interferon can also trigger infected body cells to undergo apoptosis, or programmed cell death. A dead body cell can no longer be used by viruses as the machinery for their replication, so self-destruction serves the greater good in this case.

While transfer factors, which pull the body toward Th1 immune activity, do not appear to work well for MS, there is compelling clinical evidence that drugs like Rebif, which also pull the body toward more Th1 activity, can be of benefit. They hold promise at reducing the incidence of relapses, though they do not stop the disease from progressing. For instance, in one large clinical study, 560 patients were treated with Rebif or placebo and followed for a two year period. Rebif reduced the relapse rates of patients by roughly 30% relative to placebo controls, but it did not significantly slow the progression of the disease from relapse/remitting to a more continual form.

A recent study from Spain (de Andres et al, 2007) indicates that INF, in the form of Rebif, stimulates the activity of Suppressor T-cells, a subtype of T-cells. These cells suppress the activity of B-cells, cells that make antibodies and are at the heart of what is considered the Th2 immune response. B-cells are also the cells that generate autoantibodies considered responsible for some autoimmune conditions. Thus, perhaps the synthetic INF leads to a reduction of the autoimmune response by ultimately suppressing B-cells. Further indirect evidence for the role of B-cell suppression in the clinical benefits of drugs like Rebif comes from the fact that corticosteroids are also effective at shortening the length of relapses in MS patients. Among their other effects, corticosteroids trigger cell death in B-cells, which is likely one of the ways in which they calm autoimmune responses. Given that Rebif and corticosteroids share their suppressive effect on B-cell activity, perhaps Rebif exerts some of its therapeutic benefits via this route. However, unlike corticosteroids, which only suppress the immune response, drugs like Rebif might also help the body deal with underlying infections by augmenting Th1 immunity.

Importantly, it also appears that INF can suppress the activity of the recently discovered Th17 cells, which are thought to play roles in the pathophysiology of autoimmune conditions like MS (Steinman, 2007). This could represent an additional mechanism by which INF synthetics like Rebif work.

There has been growing interest in using Low Dose Naltrexone (LDN) as immunotherapy in the treatment of MS. As the impact of LDN on the immune system is similar to that of transfer factors, it is worth discussing here. Naltrexone blocks the activation of opiate receptors, making it useful in blocking the pleasure induced via opiate abuse and in bringing one back from the brink of death following an opiate overdose. At far lower doses (5 mg vs. 50+ mg), naltrexone produces a subtle blockade of opiate receptors followed by an increase in endogenous opiate (endorphin) activity as the body attempts to reestablish homeostatis. Growing evidence suggests that this process can be of significant clinical benefit to those with a wide range of immune-related conditions, from MS to chronic Lyme and HIV. The explanation seems to rest in the fact that Natural Killer cells are spurred into action by endorphins via beta-endorphin receptors on their cell membranes. Thus, the rebound increase in endorphin activity following nightly treatment with LDN triggers increases in Natural Killer cell activity, which likely pulls the whole of the immune response in the Th1 direction and away from the autoimmune response associated with MS, perhaps by helping the body deal with intracellular pathogens.

While the underlying cause of MS is not known, recent research indicates that most sufferers of MS, upwards of 95%, test positive for active infections with HHV-6, a herpes virus that we discussed in the section on ME/CFS. If this virus is the underlying culprit, then treating patients with immune boosting drugs that target HHV-6 should help alleviate the symptoms of the condition. Transfer factors with specificity for HHV-6 are now available in supplemental form and can be taken orally. To date, no studies have been conducted to assess the effectiveness of HHV-6 transfer factor preparations against MS. Such studies would be extremely informative, as their success or failure would allow researchers to determine whether HHV-6 plays a role in the pathology underlying MS, or if its presence in MS sufferers is simply a reflection of aberrant immune function and a suscepti-bility to opportunistic infections in general.

The beneficial effect of the synthetic compound, glatira-mer acetate, against MS yields insight into the pathophysiology involved in the condition and is worth exploring here. Glatira-mer, sold as Copaxone in the US and Canada, is a combination of four amino acids found in the myelin that surrounds nerve cells. As discussed above, MS is associated with an attack on the glial cells that create myelin. During a typical immune response, cells like macrophages engulf a pathogen and present its antigen to T-cells, which then coordinate additional battles against the pathogen. Glatiramer displaces the myelin-related antigen being presented to the T-cells. As a result, the immune system is tricked into ceasing to attack the myelin. Further, the process evoked by glatiramer results in the movement of a special form of Suppressor T-cells to the brain where they suppress further immune responses toward the myelin. In clinical trials, patients receiving glatiramer experienced around a 30% reduction in episodes over a two year period. The safety profile appears to be more than satisfactory, though daily injections are required. (see Arnon and Aharoni, 2004, in the references for a review of the mechanisms from the researchers that created the compound).

In summary, MS is a condition in which the myelin sheath around the axons of neurons degenerates, thereby interfering with the ability of these cells to send signals, trigger muscle movement, carry sensory (e.g., touch) information, etc. The disorder seems to have an immune basis, but the nature of it remains unclear. Based on the available evidence, transfer factors do not seem to have much utility in treating MS. Other immunomodulators, including synthetic INF (e.g., Rebif) and low doses of opiate receptor blockers (naltrexone) do help.

At present, transfer factors aimed at specific pathogens that might underlie the disorder have not been tried. It is possible that, if specific pathogens that cause the condition are identified, transfer factors might be the best solution. It is also possible that the immune cells of primary interest in MS reside beyond the Th1/Th2 distinction. That is, the trigger might involve hypo-activity of Suppressor T-cells (Leceta et al., 2007) or hyper-activity of Th17 cells (Steinman, 2007).

Given the failure of transfer factors to improve MS, this section could have included only one brief paragraph, or not have been included at all. However, by exploring what is known and not known about the causes of MS, it is the author's hope the reader will recognize that the failure of transfer factors to improve conditions like MS likely stems from the complicated causes of the conditions rather than an inherent weakness in transfer factor therapy.

4.3 Transfer factors in the treatment of specific viruses, bacteria, mycobacteria and fungi

The conditions discussed above – cancer, ME/CFS, FM, RA and MS – are complicated conditions of poorly understood etiology. Evidence suggests that transfer factors can be of pronounced benefit for some patients with cancer or ME/CFS, and can help prevent opportunistic infections during chemotherapy. They are of less utility for those suffering from FM and

MS, most likely because transfer factors do not produce the types of changes needed to counteract the problems underlying the conditions, whatever those might be. They also hold promise in the treatment of RA.

Ultimately, the causes of these conditions are unknown. Indeed, there is incredible variability in the clinical symptoms and biological markers seen in subjects labeled with the same conditions. One patient with RA might show evidence of viral infections while others might not. Some subjects with ME/CFS exhibit evidence of insufficient Th1-mediated immune activity, including low Natural Killer cell levels, while others show normal markers of Th1 function. As such, it is incredibly difficult to determine the reasons why transfer factors work in some instances and not in others. Similar problems plague the interpretation of all clinical studies assessing the effectiveness of drugs and supplements in treating immune-related conditions with unknown causes.

As we have already seen, evidence for the effectiveness of transfer factors is most apparent when assessing their impact on individual pathogens. In the studies we examined, not all patients with ME/CFS and concomitant infections with HHV-6 or CMV exhibited improvements in clinical markers of ME/CFS, but the vast majority exhibited a resolution of their viral infections. Given the growing problem with viral infections, evidence suggesting that transfer factors are effective against viruses is extremely important from a public health standpoint. As stated by Steven Bock (2000):

> "Currently in medicine, we are seeing increased problems with viral infections, such as otitis media, measles, chronic fatigue, Epstein-Barr virus (EBV), CMV, acquired immunodeficiency syndrome (AIDS), hepatitis, and West Nile virus. We utilize treatment regimens that range from interferon to azidothymidine (AZT), riba-

virin, and relenza. However, even with all the high-tech immune weapons available, we are still losing the battle. In the treatment of viral infections, transfer factor provides a modality that works at a fundamental level."

There are several advantages to clinical studies in which transfer factors are used for specific pathogens relative to those studies involving poorly defined conditions. One is obvious – the pathogen being targeted is known, its presence can be demonstrated prior to treatment, and success can be judged by its presence or absence after the treatment. Throw in a control group and the results are even easier to interpret. A second advantage is that transfer factors can be tailor made for specific pathogens of interest. Broad spectrum transfer factors boost Th1-mediated immune activity, but there are no guarantees that the elevated immune activity will lead to pitched battles against the pathogen(s) causing a particular ailment. Transfer factors with known specificity for a pathogen elevate overall immune activity, but also direct some of it toward that particular disease causing microbe.

In this section, we will focus on studies that have examined the ability of transfer factors to help the immune system overcome specific viral, bacterial, mycobacterial and fungal infections.

Herpes viruses

There are eight known herpes viruses, including the herpes simplex viruses (HSV-1 and HSV-2), which cause herpes outbreaks on the face and genitals respectively, the varicella-zoster virus (VZV) that causes chicken pox and shingles, cyto-megalovirus (CMV), the Epstein-Barr virus (EBV) that causes mononucleosis, and the HHV-6 A&B viruses now associated with conditions like ME/CFS and MS. Research evaluating the ability of transfer factors to help the immune system overcome these viruses has yielded overwhelmingly positive results – even when broad spectrum transfer factor preparations are used. Let us take a look at a few of those studies.

Khan and colleagues (1981) examined the ability of transfer factors to prevent relapses in 16 subjects with recurrent HSV-1 (cold sores) and HSV-2 (genital) outbreaks. Patients were injected with broad spectrum transfer factors on a weekly or monthly basis. Following treatment, eight patients stopped having outbreaks altogether while the remaining eight exhibited a significant reduction in the frequency of outbreaks. Roughly half of all subjects exhibited low T-cell counts at the study onset, and all patients exhibited an increase in T-cell numbers after treatment with transfer factors.

Pizza et al (1996) reported that 44 patients suffering from recurrent HSV outbreaks – 22 with genital outbreaks and 22 with labial (face) outbreaks – responded positively to treatment with transfer factors specific to HSV-1 and HSV-2. Research from the same lab, also published in 1996 (Meduri et al, 1996), demonstrated the ability of HSV-specific transfer factors to reduce the frequency of outbreaks in those whose outbreaks occurred in the eyes.

Currently, there are several prescription drugs available that are capable of reducing the frequency and duration of HSV-1 and HSV-2 outbreaks. The active component of most such drugs is acyclovir. The drugs differ in the amount of acyclovir that they actually deliver to the body in useable form. Does acyclovir work? Absolutely. When taken daily, it reduces the frequency of outbreaks, and the outbreaks that occur are of shorter duration and lesser intensity. When taken only for acute outbreaks, they shorten their duration but have no impact on the frequency of outbreaks throughout the year. It also appears to have a satisfactory safety profile.

It seems that acyclovir does the trick by disrupting viral replication inside of infected cells. Herpes viruses insert their own DNA into the DNA of host cells, thereby using the host cells as factories to replicate the virus. Acyclovir somehow disrupts the process. However, because the drug directly targets the virus and does not modify immune function in any appreciable way, its effects are short-lasting and the drug must be taken frequently to be effective. Further, if the original infection resulted from an immune weakness of some kind, acyclovir will not help fix the underlying problems.

As discussed above, like acyclovir, transfer factors also reduce the frequency and severity of herpes outbreaks. A few studies have directly compared the efficacy of these two approaches against the viruses. Estrada-Parra and colleagues (1995) administered transfer factors to 20 patients suffering from recurrent outbreaks of HSV-1. Most patients had already been treated with acyclovir prior to their inclusion in the study. Broad spectrum transfer factors reduced both the frequency and duration of outbreaks in patients. Their observations led the authors to conclude:

> "These results suggest that, at present, TF may
> be considered the therapeutic agent of choice in
> the treatment of herpes simplex type 1 disease."

The findings of the above study are limited by the fact that no direct comparison to acyclovir was actually made. The superiority of transfer factors over acyclovir was inferred from the comparison of current treatment outcomes to the patients' prior experiences with acyclovir and other drugs.

In 1998, this same group of researchers reported findings from a study in which they directly compared the effectiveness of transfer factors and acyclovir against outbreaks of VZV, the herpes virus that causes chicken pox in kids and shingles in adults. In this study, 28 patients with acute outbreaks of shingles were given either transfer factors or acyclovir for seven days and then monitored for another 14 days. The study was double-blind, meaning that neither the doctors nor the patients knew which treatment patients received until the end of the study. Transfer factors were superior to acyclovir at shortening the duration of the outbreaks. Further, transfer factors, but not acyclovir, increased the number of Helper T-cells and improved other markers of immune function.

In addition to clinical trials, there are several reports in the literature of individual cases in which ill patients infected with herpes viruses were helped by transfer factors, usually after conventional treatments failed. Such case studies can be fascinating and suggestive, but broad conclusions cannot be drawn from them.

From Jones and colleagues (1981):

"An illness lasting for two years, with recurrent fever, rash, abdominal pain, and arthralgia, developed in a four year old boy. He was found to have a combined Epstein-Barr virus and cytomegalovirus (CMV) infection. His symptoms, CMV in his urine, and an absent in vitro lymphocyte response to CMV antigen persisted for two years. After treatment with orally administered bovine transfer factor clinical symptoms and viruria disappeared and specific immunity to CMV developed."

And from Winkelmann and colleagues (1984):

"A 29-year-old woman with a long history of immunoreactive disease—thrombocytopenic purpura, bullous pemphigoid, nephropathy, and hemolytic anemia—contracted generalized herpes zoster and varicella pneumonia. Respiratory failure requiring assisted respiration accompanied progressive chest findings. She recovered rapidly simultaneous with the administration of transfer factor from a healing herpes zoster patient. We believe that this therapy should be attempted in similar desperate circumstances."

Humans are complicated animals and are subject to confounding effects, including the placebo effect in which improvements can result simply because the patient, or doctor, expects them to occur. Lab animals are not generally subject to such confounds. Research with lab animals, like that with humans, demonstrates the powerful effects of specific transfer factors against herpes viruses. Viza et al (1986) assessed the efficacy of transfer factors in preventing the deleterious effects of HSV-1 and -2 by administering HSV-1 and -2 specific transfer factors to mice before exposing them to a normally deadly dose of the viruses. The HSV-specific transfer factor preparation protected the animals from death. Interestingly a transfer factor preparation specific to CMV rather than HSV-1 and -2 did not protect the animals from the lethal dose of HSV.

Findings from the above study reinforce the importance of using transfer factor preparations with known specificity to the disease-causing pathogen of interest whenever possible. While broad spectrum transfer factors could improve a patient's prognosis simply by boosting immune system health in general, they will be less effective against specific threats than transfer factors tailored to those threats.

Findings regarding the effectiveness of transfer factors against herpes viruses clash with claims made by GlaxoSmithKline, the makers of Valtrex, a form of the drug acyclovir. Television ads for Valtrex claim that it is the only medicine proven to reduce herpes outbreaks. Given that only drugs approved by the FDA, not supplements, can be titled "medicines" by law, this is technically true. However, science has shown that transfer factors with specificity for herpes viruses are actually superior to acyclovir in head-to-head clinical studies.

Valtrex ads point out that the drug is only for people with healthy immune systems. This is not the case with transfer factors. Transfer factors for herpes viruses improve immune markers, as has been observed in studies directly comparing acyclovir against transfer factors for herpes outbreaks, making them ideal for those with weakened immune systems.

As mentioned in the section on ME/CFS, research presented by scientists at Stanford University Medical Center suggests that valganciclovir (Valcyte) is effective at reducing symptoms of ME/CFS in patients whose illnesses began after an episode of a flu-like ailment and who tested positive for HHV-6 (Kogelnik et al, 2006). It would be of interest to examine whether adding transfer factors specific to HHV-6 would provide even further relief.

Herpes-related headaches (i.e., recurrent viral encephalitis)

When herpes infects cells near the skin, outbreaks of shingles and oral/genital herpes can occur – and *can be seen*. Given the fact that herpes viruses hide in nerve bundles and are known to come out of hiding from time to time, it is reasonable to assume that herpes outbreaks can occur wherever nerve bundles end, including below the surface, or inside the head, where there is no outward sign of infection, just pain.

Indeed, by one estimate, upwards of 1 in 10 female patients who acquire genital herpes experience excruciating head pain during the first outbreak. Kleinschmidt-DeMasters and Gilden (2001) report that several different strains of herpes viruses – including the varicella zoster virus associated with shingles, Epstein Barr virus associated with mononucleosis, HHV-6, cytomegalovirus, HSV-1 associated with oral herpes and HSV-2 associated with genital herpes – all can cause encephalitis and recurrent meningitis in outwardly healthy people. As such, herpes-related headaches could account for a large percentage of headaches suffered around the world in a given day.

Here are some comments about the experience of herpes-related headaches posted on a resource site, www.herpes-coldsores.com (content posted on November 30, 2008 and accessed January 11, 2009):

> "I have had 3 outbreaks [of herpes] in a row in the last 5 days, literally on top of the other, and yesterday I could not function due to the head pain. Down in my jaw around the back of neck and especially across the front, yes it is exactly like a cluster head ache. Nothing can touch this pain either."

Reports from people with these headaches suggest they often last for 7-14 days, in line with the length of typical herpes outbreaks.

Much of the pain that comes with these infections might actually be triggered by inflammation of the casing around the nerve bundle, which could cause large numbers of pain fibers to become irritated on their way into the spinal cord/brain and cause intense back and head pain. That scenario would explain how people could have so much pain without any apparent damage in the areas that hurt. The pain would basically be referred pain caused by inflammation of the whole nerve bundle rather than activation of the pain receptors where it seems to hurt and could explain why MRI and other scans fail to find abnormalities in the painful areas.

If a patient's recurring headaches are comorbid with herpes infections, there are good reasons to believe that herpes-specific transfer factors could reduce both the frequency and duration of such episodes. In the absence of herpes-specific transfer factors, common antivirals for herpes viruses, or readily available broad spectrum transfer factors, could help instead. As with butterbur for migraines, the benefits would be realized as fewer and shorter episodes. With herpes-related headaches, as with herpes-related oral and genital outbreaks, it should be possible to achieve long-lasting remission once the immune system finally gets the upper hand.

Yeast infections

Several studies have examined the efficacy of transfer factor preparations in treating yeast infections, particularly infections that fall into the category of Chronic Mucocutaneous Candidiasis (CMC). This category actually reflects a number of different conditions in which a patient presents with recurring or persistent yeast infections in the nails, skin or mucous membranes. These infections are typically caused by the *Candida* genus of yeast. Most patients with them share at least one thing in common – weak cell-mediated immunity against yeast of the Candida variety. This weak immunity could be specific to Candida or, as is the case with AIDS patients, could result from weakened Th1 immunity in general.

Perhaps better than anything else, transfer factors evoke or restore cell-mediated (Th1) immunity to specific pathogens. Given the faulty cell-mediated immunity to Candida in CMC patients, one would expect transfer factors to be of great benefit to those suffering from CMC. Research suggests that this is the case. In 1996, Masi and colleagues reported on a study in which they examined the efficacy of Candida-specific transfer factors at treating CMC in 15 patients. At the onset of the study, roughly 60% of patients exhibited detectable cell-mediated immune responses to Candida, as demonstrated by the Delayed Hypersensitivity Test. After treatment, that number climbed to 84%, reflecting the ability of transfer factors to transfer cell-mediated immunity. According to the authors, 14/15 patients exhibited improvements in their clinical presentation, suggesting that transfer factors are effective at treating CMC.

Yeast in the Candida genus also cause vaginal yeast infections, thrush and intestinal yeast overgrowth. The utility of transfer factors against these conditions has not been assessed.

However, logically, they should be effective. In mice, experimentally induced cell-mediated immunity to Candida seems to help the body get rid of Candida infections (Fidel et al., 1993). Hopefully, research evaluating the effectiveness of transfer factors against vaginal and intestinal yeast infections will be conducted in the near future.

Tuberculosis

Tuberculosis (TB) is caused by two types of mycobacteria (*Mycobacterium tuberculosis* and *Mycobacterium bovis*). Mycobacteria, also called mycoplasma, do not have cell walls like normal bacteria. This allows them to evade detection by the immune system and to hide inside of healthy body cells, including immune cells. Mycobacteria, unlike viruses, are susceptible to some antibiotics. In the case of TB, the mycobacterial infections have traditionally been treated with long-term (6-9 month) therapy with three or four antibiotics used in combination.

In the spring of 2007, the American public was reminded that highly drug resistant strains of the TB mycobacterium now exist. The news came via reports that an American lawyer traveled overseas on a passenger plane despite advice against the trip from the CDC. The report turned out to be inaccurate and the patient had a more treatable form of TB. However, it generated renewed interest in TB and the risks it can pose.

As an indication that drug companies view treatments for TB as potentially lucrative, GlaxoSmithKline currently (January, 2009) lists finding better ways to battle the "white plague" (TB) as one of its future aims (www.gsk.com).

A vaccine, known as BCG, exists for TB. However, due to the low incidence of TB in the U.S., it is not currently administered.

The initial discovery of transfer factor by Dr. H.S. Lawrence was made when he transferred cell-mediated immunity from a patient that had been exposed to TB to one that had not been exposed to TB. His initial findings have been replicated, with great success.

Rates of TB have dropped around the world, with the exception of hotspots in Africa, Eastern Europe, Russia and among the aging in Japan, where the disease seems to be re-emerging in those infected during their youth. In the event of a resurgence of TB, even highly drug resistant strains, transfer factors should be able to protect naïve subjects from infection, or at least minimize the severity. They should also hold promise in the treatment of active infections, including those unresponsive to current antibiotic therapy.

Rocklin (1975) reports on a single patient with TB:

> "The patient had not responded clinically or bacteriologically after 7 1/2 months of antituberculous therapy, although the organism was shown to be sensitive in vitro to the drugs she was receiving. She received 6 doses of dialysable transfer factor over a 3-month period and during this time she responded clinically, bacteriologically and roentgenographically."

At the very least, it should be comforting to know that there are options for the management of TB beyond traditional antibiotic therapy.

Human Immunodeficiency Virus (HIV)

Since first being diagnosed in 1983, infections with HIV have claimed the lives of more than 20 million people worldwide. HIV is one of a category of viruses called retroviruses. HIV consists of a protein ball containing some genetic information in the form of RNA. The virus also contains enzymes capable of converting the RNA into DNA and then splicing the DNA into that of the host's cells. Once this step is completed, the host's cells begin making replicas of the HIV. Eventually, the host's cells are used to secrete the virus into the extracellular fluid, where it can infect other cells.

Despite widespread reports associating HIV with homosexuality, the virus is spread through male-to-male sexual contact in only about 40% of cases. Thirty percent of new HIV cases result from heterosexual contact while 25% stem from sharing contaminated needles. Other cases are acquired by offspring during gestation.

The virus is spread by contact with mucosal membranes, such as those in the vagina, penis, rectum and – rarely – the mouth. It appears that the virus attaches to immune cells in these mucous membranes, which then carry the virus to lymph nodes where the real infection begins.

HIV primarily infects Helper T-cells. It attaches to the membranes of these cells and then injects the viral payload into them. The virus incapacitates the immune system by taking over these cells, which are like air traffic controllers that direct immune responses. Without sufficient, functional Helper T-cells, the immune system simply cannot wage an effective battle against HIV or other pathogens. In addition to infecting Helper T-cells, the virus also infects Natural Killer cells and macrophages. It appears that macrophages are capable of carrying around large loads of the virus without dying, meaning that they become repositories for this insidious threat and deliver it to unsuspecting Helper T-cells throughout the body.

The pathogenesis of the HIV infection, and its progression to full-blown Acquired Immune Deficiency Syndrome (AIDS), is captured in the following summary from the National Institutes of Health (NIH, 2004):

> "Untreated HIV disease is characterized by a gradual deterioration of immune function. Most notably, crucial immune cells called CD4 positive (CD4+) T cells are disabled and killed during the typical course of infection... A healthy,

uninfected person usually has 800 to 1,200 CD4+ T cells per cubic millimeter (mm3) of blood. During untreated HIV infection, the number of these cells in a person's blood progressively declines. When the CD4+ T cell count falls below 200/mm3, a person becomes particularly vulnerable to the opportunistic infections and cancers that typify AIDS, the end stage of HIV disease... Most scientists think that HIV causes AIDS by directly inducing the death of CD4+ T cells or interfering with their normal function, and by triggering other events that weaken a person's immune function. For example, the network of signaling molecules that normally regulates a person's immune response is disrupted during HIV disease, impairing a person's ability to fight other infections... Immunosuppression by HIV is confirmed by the fact that medicines, which interfere with the HIV lifecycle, preserve CD4+ T cells and immune function as well as delay clinical illness."

In other words, most of the damage done by HIV comes from the infection and death of Helper T-cells, though some researchers believe that the drop in Helper T-cells occurs due to exhaustion of the immune system while trying to fight HIV. Regardless, the drop in Helper T-cells impairs the ability of the body to mount Th1-mediated immune responses. Eventually, the body's ability to fight infections is suppressed to the point that the body simply succumbs to infections and cancers.

HIV is a complicated virus, and one capable of mutating quickly. This makes it notoriously difficult to treat or to prevent with vaccines. When left untreated, HIV infection typically progresses to full-blown AIDS over 10-12 years, though the progression can be markedly faster or slower depending on factors like the overall health of the individual and the cleanliness of the surrounding environment.

A long list of steps is involved in the replication and spread of HIV, offering scientists numerous options for targeting the virus with drugs. Some drugs block the ability of the virus to fuse with Helper T-cells. Others aim at preventing the insertion of the HIV genetic material into the DNA of the host. Most of the antiviral drugs approved by the FDA for the treatment of HIV work by interfering with viral replication.

At its core, the pathogenesis of HIV and its progression to AIDS involves a debilitating attack on cells that comprise the Th1-mediated immune response, particularly Helper T-cells. It seems logical to expect that transfer factors could be powerful adjuvants in the treatment of HIV given their ability to trigger increased levels of Helper T-cells, as well as Cytotoxic T-cells, Natural Killer cells and macrophages. While transfer factors alone might not be able to prop up immune system health sufficiently to defeat HIV, it sure seems that they should be able to at least slow the progression of HIV to AIDS by keeping Helper T-cell levels elevated above the critical threshold that leads to AIDS.

Currently, only a few studies have examined the utility of transfer factors in the treatment of HIV/AIDS, but the available data are promising. Carey et al (1987) assessed the impact of transfer factors from healthy controls on immune system function in nine patients with HIV infections that had progressed to full-blown AIDS. They concluded that:

> "..administration of transfer factor to patients with AIDS resulted in partial immune reconstitution. Further studies are indicated to examine the clinical efficacy of this immune response modifier in the treatment of AIDS."

In 1996, Giancarlo Pizza and colleagues reported on a study in which they administered HIV specific transfer factors, in an oral preparation, to 25 patients infected with HIV. They noted clinical improvements or a stabilization of clinical markers in 20/25 patients. Interestingly, not all patients exhibited an increase in Helper T-cells during treatment with transfer factors. Cell counts increased in 11/25 patients but decreased in 11/25 patients.

The HIV virus has the ability to disable, or turn off, Helper T-cells. Thus, while the cells show up in cell counts, they are essentially useless. In 12/14 patients with this condition, known as *anergy*, Helper T-cells became active again during transfer factor therapy. The authors concluded that:

> "These preliminary observations suggest that oral HIV-specific TF administration, in association with antiviral drugs, is well tolerated and seems beneficial to AIDS patients, thus warranting further investigation."

That same year, Pizza and colleagues (Raise et al, 1996) reported the results of a study in which they directly compared groups receiving standard antiviral therapy to those receiving combined antiviral therapy and HIV-specific transfer factors. Patients received either Zidovudine alone or in combination with transfer factors. Those receiving the Zidovudine-transfer factor combination exhibited a larger increase in Cytotoxic T-cell counts and in the levels of interleukin-2, a critical immune messenger that promotes the genesis of T-cells and promotes the Th1 immune response in general. Interestingly, however, there were no differences between the groups regarding actual levels of Helper T-cells.

A 2002 report from Russian scientists also suggests that transfer factors could play an important role in the management of HIV (Granitov et al, 2002). The researchers examined immune cell counts in HIV patients administered a commercially available oral transfer factor supplement. Fifteen patients were treated with transfer factors alone. Ten patients in a control group were treated with common antivirals for HIV but not transfer factors. Treatment lasted for only seven days and immune measurements were taken one week later.

The majority of subjects in the transfer factor group exhibited increased levels of Helper T-cells and Cytotoxic T-cells. The pattern of cytokine release was altered in transfer factor-treated subjects in a way that facilitates Th1 immune activity. Levels of circulating immune complexes, which reflect the combination of an antibody and an antigen, were reduced to normal levels in 10 of 15 subjects. In the control group, positive changes were as likely to occur as negative changes. In the words of the authors (Granitov et al, 2002):

> "We conclude that transfer factors therapy considerably improves the immune status of HIV-infected patients and can be recommended in combating the pathogenesis of the disease. Further studies are needed to determine optimal therapy, the necessity to repeat courses of the treatment and the frequency of therapy needed."

Two recent studies from researchers at the Center for Biological Research in Havana, Cuba, suggest that transfer factors are capable of directly interfering with HIV replication (Ojeda et al, 2000; Fernandez-Ortega et al, 2004). If the mechanisms underlying this effect are identified, it might be possible to formulate transfer factor preparations with heightened activity against HIV replication. Such preparations could prove extremely useful when combined with other antivirals currently used in the battle against HIV.

In the case of HIV and other disorders involving too much Th2 immune activity and not enough Th1 function, the benefits of transfer factors would likely be extended by co-administration of something like low doses of naltrexone (LDN), discussed earlier in the chapter. The mild opiate receptor blockade caused by small amounts of naltrexone gives way to a compensatory increase in the body's levels of endorphins. It turns out that Natural Killer cells are spurred into action by the binding of endorphins to beta-endorphin receptors. By using small amounts of this very safe drug, Natural Killer cell activity is augmented. It is unclear what happens next, but an overall shift in immune function toward the cell-mediated side is likely triggered by the increased Natural Killer cell activity. This process could help the body wrest some control away from HIV and start fighting back. A clinical trial of LDN for HIV is currently underway in Mali, led by wife and husband team Jaquelyn McCandless, MD and Jack Zimmerman, PhD.

Given their safety profile, their ability to help stave off opportunistic infections, their impact on T-cell levels and cytokine release profiles, and their low cost, transfer factors should be carefully considered for HIV/AIDS patients, particularly those with poor access to other treatment options.

Transfer factors and HIV vaccines

Hindsight is not quite 20-20 when it comes to drug development or science in general. It is always tempting to connect historical dots to create best fitting lines – ones that suggest linearity in progress and often ignore false starts and dead ends. In the case of vaccine development, it seems HIV vaccine researchers reached a dead end in 2008. One ultimately caused by a false start caused by a false logical premise. HIV is not a disease best dealt with through vaccines. In essence, vaccines, at least as designed now, cannot trigger cell-mediated immunity to HIV, which is what is needed to beat it. Vaccines are good, however, at triggering antibody-mediated immunity, which is helpful in some cases but makes conditions ripe for infections with sneaky viruses like HIV.

HIV is a virus that functions in ways requiring a great deal more Th1, cell-mediated, immune activity to defeat than other viruses. It climbs inside macrophages near the surface of the body and sneaks a ride to lymph nodes where it infects Th1 cells and the disease sets in. This leaves very little time for antibodies to do their job. Indeed, a vaccine-induced increase in antibody-mediated immune activity would lead to a temporary reduction in resources going to cell-mediated immune activity, perhaps making it even easier for HIV to get behind the gates.

Such a scenario could explain why, in 2008, the combined Merck-NIH vaccine for HIV, V520, was found to *increase* the risk of HIV infection rather than decrease it. The aim of the vaccine was to evoke, somehow, cell-mediated immunity to HIV. Here is an explanation of the logic from a recent manuscript by the author of the current book (White, 2008a):

> "V520 consists of a deactivated cold virus, in this case adenovirus-5, modified to express proteins associated with the internal contents of the HIV virus rather than proteins located on the virus' shell... The hope was that V520 would trigger CD8+ Cytotoxic T-cells to recognize healthy body cells infected with the internal components of HIV and destroy them. In other words, the hope was to evoke, somehow, cell-mediated immunity to HIV. This did not happen"

The vaccine backfired, probably because the very nature of vaccines makes them best at triggering antibody-mediated, not cell-mediated, immunity. Those previously exposed to the cold virus used in the vaccine, particularly if they were uncircumcised males, were at increased risk of HIV infection. Logically, this suggests that the vaccine inadvertently caused suppression of the exact immune response, the cell-mediated one, that it tried to augment. Again, from White (2008a):

"It is quite likely that vaccines like Merck's V520 actually give HIV a head start by hobbling the subjects' cell-mediated immunity. This hypothesis gets support from the fact that subjects previously exposed to the adenovirus-5 cold virus used in the vaccine were at greater risk of HIV infection after vaccination with V520. Presumably, those previously exposed to the virus would exhibit a stronger antibody-mediated response, and thus a more dampened cell-mediated response, upon re-exposure to the cold virus."

A recent study provides support for the above hypothesis. Benlahrech and colleagues (2009) reported that re-exposure to the adenovirus in previously exposed subjects triggered an increase in the expression of adenovirus-specific CD4 Helper T-cells and the migration of these cells to the mucosa where they serve as additional targets for HIV infection.

In the wake of the failure of V520, some researchers suggested that the potential value of cell-mediated approaches to HIV prevention, in general, should now be in question. In a letter to the editor of the medical journal, *The Lancet*, which published the results of the Step Study, the study that assessed V520, the author of the current book makes the case that the failure of the Step Study says very little about the value of cell-mediated approaches for dealing with HIV. Here is an excerpt from the letter (White, 2009):

"It is vital that discussions of the Step Study's failure and about future directions for HIV vaccine research are not predicated on the mistaken assumption that the Step Study represents a perfect test of the utility of cell-mediated approaches for HIV prevention. It does not. Indeed, it seems likely that the design of the vaccine used in the study, rather than its intended purpose of evoking cell-mediated immunity, could be at the center of the Step Study's failure."

The letter does not mention transfer factors but they remain the logical means of assessing the value of cell-mediated immune approaches for preventing HIV. Could HIV-specific transfer factors serve the purpose of HIV vaccines? Earlier in the chapter, we explored the utility of transfer factors for treating HIV infections. Below is an excerpt from White (2008a) exploring the potential use of transfer factors for HIV prevention:

"If HIV-specific transfer factors were given to subjects before exposure to HIV, the odds of contracting the virus should go down considerably, and without evoking an entirely abnormal, and unnecessary, surge of antibody-mediated immune activity. Theoretically, HIV-specific transfer factors extracted from cow colostrum or egg yolks and taken orally would program the cell-mediated immune pathway to hunt down and destroy cells infected with HIV. One portion of the transfer factor molecule would bind to antigens on the surface of infected cells and another would bind to CD4+ Helper T-cells, triggering them to mount an attack. If the body has such instructions before it is exposed to HIV, it might be capable of keeping the virus at bay and preventing it from taking hold."

In short, it is possible that transfer factors could serve the purpose of immunizing subjects against HIV better than

HIV vaccines can. At present, the most advanced vaccines have either failed or increased the odds of contracting HIV. Even the legendary vaccine researcher, Jonas Salk, failed at creating an effective HIV vaccine (Gorman and Park, 1995). No prospective studies have assessed the ability of HIV-specific transfer factors to prevent HIV infection, though research does suggest they are useful during HIV treatment. Hopefully, their ability to prevent infections will be assessed at some point in the near future.

Unexpected evidence of the importance of cell-mediated immunity in the fight against HIV

In the fall of 2008, an American patient living in Germany and suffering with both leukemia and HIV was apparently cured of both conditions following a bone marrow transplant from a unique donor. The donor possessed a very rare genetic variation that makes it difficult for HIV to enter into his healthy cells. In other words, the genetic anomaly conveys inherent cell-mediated immunity to HIV. In essence, by transplanting bone marrow from this particular donor to the HIV positive patient, the patient developed a new immune system capable of fending off HIV.

Following the report, White (2008b) wrote an article published on the website *Medical News Today* examining what the finding suggests about the role of cell-mediated immunity in HIV treatment and prevention. Transfer factors are offered as a logical alternative to bone marrow transplants for reprogramming the immune system to deal with HIV. Below is an excerpt:

> "Bone marrow transplants might not be the most efficacious, or comfortable, means of rebuilding an immune system that can contend with HIV. However, there are other means of reprogramming the immune system, and without putting the patient's life at greater risk. Vaccines offer

one such approach, but one thus far proven ineffective and even detrimental for those at risk of contracting HIV. Vaccines reprogram the immune system by triggering it to generate antibodies to proteins, or antigens, on the surface of viruses... While antibodies can provide protection before a virus infiltrates host cells, transfer factors are needed to lead the immune system to host cells once they are infected...More research would be helpful, but that already done indicates that one can literally transfer immunity to infectious agents using this technology, and that transfer factors are quite helpful in fighting infections once they have set in. HIV, along with unrelated intracellular pathogens like Lyme, are able to suppress the cell-mediated pathway while simultaneously activating the antibody-mediated pathway. This enables them to hide. Transfer factors for those specific agents trigger the immune system to go searching for them and, in the process, pull the body away from the antibody mediated response and in the right direction."

The existence of a genetic anomaly that allows people to beat HIV by expressing inherent cell-mediated immunity to it provides compelling reasons to believe that cell-mediated immune approaches to HIV prevention *could* work. Presently, transfer factors offer the best possible means of assessing the true utility of cell-mediated immunity in the fight against the disease.

Helicobacter pylori and ulcers

Ulcers, or holes, in the stomach and intestines are common causes of abdominal pain. Once thought due mainly to stress and poor dietary choices, current thinking pins the problem on infections with the bacterium, *Helicobacter pylori* (H. pylori). According to the CDC, more than 90% of duodenal (intestinal) ulcers are caused by H. pylori, as are around 80% of gastric (stomach) ulcers. Eight strategies are approved by the FDA for the treatment of ulcers, all involving a combination of acid reducers and antibiotics.

A 2004 report from the Russian Ministry of Health summarizes their findings from clinical studies assessing the utility of transfer factors in treating H. pylori related ulcers. While imperfect (no true control group), the findings are of interest here and suggest transfer factors could be a promising treatment approach for ulcers associated with H. pylori.

Thirty-five patients with duodenal ulcers associated with H. pylori were divided into two groups. Group One (15 patients) received omeprazole (sold in the U.S. as Prilosec) and two antibiotics – amoxycillin and clarythromycin – for 10 days. Group Two received the above drug cocktail for 10 days along with a commercial transfer factor preparation for a full 30 days. Patients in the transfer factor group recovered sooner and exhibited improvements in Natural Killer cell and T-cell levels relative to those in the standard treatment group. Antibiotics alone eradicated H. pylori infections in 73% of subjects. In the antibiotics + transfer factors group, H. pylori was eradicated in 95% of patients.

Collectively, the data suggest transfer factors could play an important and effective role in treating ulcers related to infections with H. pylori.

4.4 Using transfer factors to prevent large-scale outbreaks of bacteria and viruses

Transfer factors are so-named because they can transfer cell-mediated immunity from host to host. This ability is highlighted by the research with TB discussed above. How do they do so?

Transfer factors seem to prime the body for battle against intracellular pathogens, like viruses, mycobacteria and CWD-bacteria, and help quash infections before they can take root. Transfer factors turn non-immune-related white blood cells into immune-related white blood cells and stimulate the birth of new Helper and Cytotoxic T-cells, Natural Killer cells and macrophages. After stimulating an increase in T-cell counts, transfer factors orient these new T-cells toward a target, presumably by influencing the nature of the antigen receptors expressed by the cells. Further, by binding to antigens on infected body cells, transfer factors paint infected cells for destruction by Cytotoxic T-cells.

In essence, supplemental transfer factors allow the naïve person to skip the immune response that leads to the creation of transfer factors during an immune battle. Transfer factors transfer "memory" for immune battles of the past, no matter in which host those battles originally took place. As far as the transfer factor recipient's immune system is concerned, it has already been exposed to the pathogen, and thus reacts promptly if the pathogen ever enters the body. By preparing the immune system for a pathogen before it enters the body, transfer factors remove the element of surprise critical to infestation by infectious agents and prevent cellular invasion by viruses, mycobacteria and CWD-bacteria.

Let us look at an interesting example in which the ability of transfer factors to transfer immunity was used to protect patients from contracting an illness. In 1980, Steele and colleagues used transfer factors in an effort to immunize young leukemia patients against chicken pox, caused by VZV. In the words of the authors:

> "Sixty-one patients with leukemia and no immunity to chickenpox were given dialyzable

transfer factor or placebo and followed for 12 to 30 months in a double-blind trial designed to examine the clinical efficacy of transfer factor. Sixteen patients in the transfer-factor group and 15 in the placebo group were exposed to varicella zoster, and most of them had a rise in antibody titer. Chickenpox developed in 13 of 15 exposed patients in the placebo group but in only one of 16 in the transfer-factor group."

Thus, when patients with leukemia and no resistance to chicken pox are treated with transfer factors for the chicken pox virus, almost everyone develops immunity to the virus. Compelling evidence that transfer factors are able to transfer immunity.

Given the ability of transfer factors to protect non-exposed patients from contracting infections, and the ability to custom make transfer factors for any identifiable pathogen, they could prove invaluable in the prevention of wide-spread, perhaps even pandemic, infections.

4.5 Summary

Research strongly suggests that transfer factors are effective for helping the body beat an array of disease states that involve faulty or overloaded immune function. Transfer factors extracted from human white blood cells are difficult and expensive to make, and are not available to the public. However, products containing transfer factors derived from cow colostrums and chicken eggs are available. In the next chapter, we will discuss the use of transfer factor supplements and examine some of the caveats.

Chapter 5

Availability and use of transfer factors

Transfer factors are tiny molecules that educate the immune system about threats from foreign invaders, particularly those that cause intracellular infections. They were discovered in 1949, but the discovery caused only quiet celebration as the technology needed to produce large quantities of purified transfer factors for disease treatment and prevention did not exist.

Until recently, researchers interested in assessing the effectiveness of transfer factors utilized a strategy similar to that originally utilized by the discoverer, Dr. H. Sherwood Lawrence. White blood cells from a host, preferably one that had been exposed to the pathogen of interest, were harvested and the Dialyzable Leukocyte Extract from the cells was injected into the target patient.

Truly impressive strides have been made in the past two decades toward creating a protocol for generating highly purified transfer factor preparations. Technological advances have rendered the use of human white blood cells on a study-by-study basis unnecessary. This should allow for rapid advances in the development of standardized protocols for utilizing transfer factors in disease treatment and prevention.

Researchers have taken advantage of the discovery that transfer factors are present in colostrum, the first fluid released from a breast after childbirth. This is true in humans, cows, and other mammals. They are also present inside of chicken eggs. When ingested by the offspring, transfer factors program Helper T-cells and stimulate the birth of Natural Killer cells, Cytotoxic T-cells and macrophages.

Using cow colostrum and chicken eggs as the source of transfer factors allows researchers to make specific transfer factors for pathogens ranging from different strains of herpes viruses to the bacterium that causes Lyme disease. This is done by exposing the host cow or chicken to the pathogen before the transfer factors are extracted from the colostrum or eggs. The ability to obtain transfer factors from colostrum and eggs is a remarkable development with the potential to significantly alter the future of disease treatment and prevention.

Now that transfer factors can be purified and are available in supplement form, the question must be asked — should they be considered supplements, which can be sold directly to the public, or drugs that should require prescriptions and only be sold by pharmaceutical companies?

5.1 Transfer factors made from cow colostrum and chicken eggs are supplements by law

The Dietary Supplement Health and Education Act (DSHEA) of 1994 lays out the rules regarding supplement creation, sales and marketing. Under this act, Congress defines dietary supplements as follows:

"A dietary supplement is a product taken by mouth that contains a 'dietary ingredient' intended to supplement the diet. The 'dietary ingredients' in these products may include: vitamins, minerals, herbs or other botanicals, amino acids, and substances such as enzymes, organ tissues, glandulars, and metabolites. Dietary supplements can also be extracts or concentrates, and may be found in many forms such as tablets, capsules, softgels, gelcaps, liquids, or powders. They can also be in other forms, such as a bar, but if they are, information on their label must not represent the product as a conventional food or a sole item of a meal or diet. Whatever their form may be, DSHEA places dietary supplements in a special category under the general umbrella of 'foods,' not drugs, and requires that every supplement be labeled a dietary supplement."

This next part is very important.

"A product sold as a dietary supplement and promoted on its label or in labeling* as a treatment, prevention or cure for a specific disease or condition would be considered an unapproved—and thus illegal—drug. To maintain the product's status as a dietary supplement, the label and labeling must be consistent with the provisions in the Dietary Supplement Health and Education Act (DSHEA) of 1994.

*Labeling refers to the label as well as accompanying material that is used by a manufacturer to promote and market a specific product.

Products containing transfer factors are dietary supplements and must be labeled as such. They are made from food products – cow milk and chicken eggs. They act by boosting the immune system in specific ways so that the immune system can help the body heal itself. They are not drugs that directly attack diseases or turn the immune response off.

There have been cases in which companies have touted the medicinal benefits of transfer factors too strongly and crossed the line between how drugs and supplements can be marketed. In those cases, the FDA, following procedures, sends letters detailing the specific offenses and requires that the language representing the products is changed accordingly. In some cases, the FDA has stopped the production and sale of transfer factors due to the failure of the companies to comply with FDA rules.

Portions of the text from two letters sent by the FDA to companies marketing transfer factors can be found below. Names of the companies have been excluded. The first letter, on the following page, lays out both the concerns that the FDA has about marketing related to the products mentioned, as well as clearly articulating what separates supplements from drugs in the eyes of the law. Supplements can help the body overcome diseases indirectly by boosting the ability of an organ system to do the job it already does. This is known as a *structure/function* claim. Even if supplements are effective at helping the body deal with diseases, companies still have to be quite careful that they do not overextend the claims of benefit to suggest that the supplement, by itself, plays a role in the "treatment" of a disease. Subtle regulations, but rules ultimately aimed at keeping the public safe.

LETTER 1 (1 of 1)

NOV 1 2004
Ref. No. CL-04-HFS-810-108

Dear Mr. ---:

This is to advise you that the Food and Drug Administration
(FDA) has reviewed your web site at the Internet address
http://www.----.com/--- and has determined that the products
"---" "---," and "---" are promoted for conditions that
cause the products to be drugs under section 201(g)(1) of
the Federal Food, Drug, and Cosmetic Act (the Act) [21 USC
§ 321(g)(1)]. The therapeutic claims on your web site
establish that the products are drugs because they are
intended for use in the cure, mitigation, treatment, or
prevention of disease. The marketing of these products with
these claims violates the Act...

Many of these products may be legally marketed as dietary
supplements if claims about diagnosis, cure, mitigation,
treatment, or prevention of disease are removed from the
promotional materials and the products otherwise comply
with all applicable provisions of the Act and FDA regulations...

Under the Act, as amended by the Dietary Supplement Health
and Education Act, dietary supplements may be legally
marketed with truthful and non-misleading claims to affect
the structure or function of the body (structure/function
claims), if certain conditions are met. However, claims
that dietary supplements are intended to prevent, diagnose,
mitigate, treat, or cure disease (disease claims), except-
ing health claims authorized for use by FDA, cause the
products to be drugs. The intended use of a product may be
established through product labels and labeling, catalogs,
brochures, audio and videotapes, Internet sites, or other
circumstances surrounding the distribution of the product.
FDA has published a final rule intended to clarify the
distinction between structure/function claims and disease
claims. This document is available on the Internet at
<http://vm.cfsan.fda.gov/~lrd/fr000106.html> (codified at
21 C.F.R. 101.93(g)).

Sincerely yours,
---,
Director, Division of Dietary Supplement Programs

The letter on the following page represents another notice from the FDA to a company selling transfer factors in which the agency is concerned that the company is marketing its products too aggressively and blurring the line between supplements and drugs. In this case, it seems the FDA is justified in their concerns. The company does, in fact, make broad claims about the utility of transfer factors in disease treatment.

Clearly, the FDA takes the issue of how supplements are marketed very seriously. We, the general public, should be grateful for that in most cases. Fortunately, transfer factors fit squarely into the supplement category. They are derived from food stuff (milk and eggs) and work by helping the body, the immune system in particular, function more effectively. They do not attack diseases directly and are only capable of acting by exerting effects on the immune system itself. The same is true of supplements that help the body avoid or overcome heart disease by strengthening the heart, or supplements that help slow the progression of age-related dementia by strengthening the health of the brain. Transfer factors are made by the body and normally do not exist outside of it. Thus, adding more transfer factors to the body is the perfect example of supplementation.

The purpose of including details regarding the distinction between drugs and supplements, and providing evidence that transfer factors are supplements, is simply to raise awareness that transfer factors could simply disappear if companies selling them do not remain vigilant about their marketing. Fortunately, transfer factors fit snuggly into the supplement category and should be available to the public indefinitely.

LETTER 2 (1 of 2)

WARNINGLETTER
June 2, 2005
CBER-05-O18

Dear Ms. ---:

The Food and Drug Administration (FDA) has reviewed your website at Internet address: http://www.----.com and has determined that your "transfer factor" products, derived from bovine colostrum, are being promoted for conditions that cause the products to be drugs under section 201(g) of the Federal Food, Drug, and Cosmetic Act (the Act) [21 USC321(g)] and/or biological products, as defined in section 351(i) ofthe Public Health Service Act (PHSAct) [42 USC262(i)].

Your transfer factor products, including ---, ---, ---, --- , ---, ---, ---, and ---, are considered drugs and/or biological products because the therapeutic claims, as shown on your website, establish their intended use as such. In describing your transfer factor products, your website includes the following claims:

"Transfer factor has consistently been effective in the prevention and treatment of viral infections."

"For acute onset of symptoms [from Herpes Simplex Virus and Varicella-Zoster Virus], one can expect an immediate response."

"The end product contains the important immune-supporting activities from a number of transfer factors including those for HHV-6, Epstein Barr Virus (EBV), Cytomegalovirus(CMV), Herpes Simplex Virus (HSV), and Herpes Zoster Virus (HZV)."

"Patients with a variety of conditions have tried our products, including chronic fatigue syndrome (CFS), fibromyalgia (FM), Gulf War syndrome, patients with post-Lyme symptoms (CFS or FM symptoms after Lyme disease), multiple sclerosis (MS), cancer, fever blisters/genital herpes, shingles, and other neurologic conditions and HIV patients."

LETTER 2 (2 of 2)

WARNINGLETTER
June 2, 2005
CBER-05-018

In addition, we note that your transfer factor products appear to be the same as products for which ---, Inc. was criminally convicted of marketing without a license. Specifically, the Internet websites http://www.---.com and http://www.---.com indicate that you obtain your transfer factor products from ---, LTD and that ---, LTD manufactures those transfer factor products using a patented process developed by ---, Inc. involving the isolation of transfer factors from the colostrum of cattle that have been injected with human viruses

In 2004, ---, Inc. was prosecuted by the federal government for using that patented process to manufacture transfer factor products like yours that were unapproved new drugs and unlicensed biological products, and for distributing those products into interstate commerce without a biologics license in effect. Please be advised that the company pled guilty to violation of Title 18 USC, section 371 (conspiracy) and was ordered to pay fines; euthanize the injected cattle, and abandon all colostrum previously seized by the FDA.

You should take prompt action to correct the violations noted above. Failure to correct these violations promptly may result in regulatory action such as seizure and/or injunction without further notice.

Please notify this office in writing within 15 working days ofreceipt ofthis letter of any steps you have taken or will take to correct the noted violations and to prevent their recurrence. If corrective action cannot be completed within 15 working days, state the reason for the delay and the time within which the corrections will be completed.

Sincerly,

---,
Director Office of Compliance and Biologics Quality

5.2 The size of transfer factors and their absorption following oral administration

Transfer factors, growth hormones, and other important constituents of colostrum are swallowed by infants and absorbed intact via the digestive system. However, the digestive systems of newborns are not complete, creating a window of opportunity for getting these things in. Many of these constituents would not be absorbed into the body if taken by adults. This raises the question – Do transfer factors get absorbed when taken orally?

Most of the research on transfer factors conducted over the past 50 years has involved the injection of extracts from white blood cells, though many studies utilized oral preparations with great success. As we have discussed, supplemental products containing transfer factors can now be purchased in capsules. Of import is whether the short-chains of amino acids that comprise transfer factors are absorbed into the body intact following oral administration or are broken down during digestion. The technological advances that have allowed these immune boosters to be made and sold in powdered form and taken orally are only valuable if the end product gets into the body and becomes bioavailable.

How big are transfer factors? Nobody knows for sure. In 2000, Kirkpatrick wrote the following:

> "To date, neither the primary structures nor the mechanisms of action of transfer factors have been identified. However, recent studies have shown that transfer factors can be purified to a high degree of homogeneity and that the purified transfer factors are proteinaceous and immunologically specific."

In other words, transfer factors are thought to be protein-like, with each different type of transfer factor conveying different effects on immune system activity.

Proteins are chains of amino acids. In healthy people, proteins are not absorbed directly into the body from the gastrointestinal tract. They are first broken down into shorter chains of amino acids called tripeptides (three amino acids together), dipeptides (a pair of amino acids), or single amino acids by enzymes called proteases and peptidases. While two or three amino acids might not sound like a lot, some important peptides in the body are, in fact, that short. Glutathione, an antioxidant, and thyrotropin releasing hormone, a hormone central to thyroid functioning, are only three amino acids long. Glatiramer acetate, a relatively new treatment for MS discussed in Chapter 4, consists of only four amino acids.

As discussed in Chapter 3, Kirkpatrick and colleagues discovered that, no matter how different various transfer factors might be, they all share a conserved sequence of amino acids. This conserved sequence is probably what allows transfer factors to bind to Helper T-cells and direct their activity. Additional amino acids in the chain, perhaps along with RNA, carry instructions specific to each type of transfer factor and/or allow the transfer factor to bind to particular antigens.

It appears that the conserved sequence itself is longer than three amino acids in length. In fact, it appears to be 10 amino acids in length. Kirkpatrick and colleagues did not examine the length of the active components of the transfer factor molecules. However, a guess about their length can be made based on the fact that transfer factors are thought to have a molecular weight of about 6000 Daltons (Da). For reference, tryptophan is the heaviest amino acid at 204.22 Da. Thus, if the active component of transfer factors were made exclusively from tryptophan, which they are not, a 6000 Da molecule would contain around 30 amino acids, much longer than the chains typically absorbed through the gut in healthy people. In their patent for extracting transfer factors from colostrum and egg yolks, Hennen and Lisonbee (2002) suggest that transfer factors could consist of 45 amino acids or more.

Regardless of the size of transfer factors, the evidence indicates that at least some percentage of oral transfer factors gets absorbed. How they are absorbed, how much is absorbed, and what percentage of the doses become bioavailable are not known at present. But there is little doubt that they get into the body and affect immune system activity. The evidence for this comes from published research in which oral preparations were used and their affects on the body measured, and from anecdotal evidence from case studies and the mild flu-like symptoms that oral transfer factors evoke upon initial treatment.

Kirkpatrick presented the most direct evidence available for the absorption of transfer factors in a 1996 manuscript. He and his colleagues measured Delayed-Type Hypersensitivity in mice given transfer factors under the skin or directly into the stomach. Transfer factors transferred immunity via both routes. They also measured immune markers after oral administration to humans and found increased levels of INFγ, a cytokine produced only by Th1-related Helper T-cells, Cytotoxic T-cells and Natural Killer cells.

In short, regardless of their size, oral transfer factors do get into the body and exert effects on immune-related activity.

5.3 Are they safe?

Based on the literature, transfer factors appear to be very safe – even when injected – with few adverse reactions reported in any of the 600+ clinical studies in which they have been used. Because of their small size, they do not appear to evoke any sort of immune response directed *at* them. In other words, the immune system does not attack transfer factors. However, transfer factors are quite capable of activating the immune system. They increase the release of inflammatory Th1 cytokines and strengthen Th1 immune activity in general. Many users experience mild flu-like symptoms at some point in the first month of treatment. This is generally taken as a good sign – an indication that the immune system is working.

There are anecdotal reports of clinicians administering extremely large doses to themselves and/or their patients. Only mild symptoms of immune activation have been reported.

For those with immune-related conditions, symptoms of illness often worsen before improving after transfer factor administration. This has traditionally been seen as part of the healing process. If a person feels ill because their immune system is chronically activated yet incapable of destroying the disease causing agent, then bolstering the immune system so that it can make a push to get rid of the pathogen is certain to make some people feel more ill on their way to feeling better. This is one of the paradoxical effects of recovery from chronic viral or bacterial illnesses for some people — feeling better and worse at the same time. Symptoms of the disease, including psychological symptoms, can all be exacerbated on the path to recovery. It is wise to schedule the onset of any such treatment as far from major obligations as possible just in case.

The tendency for symptoms to worsen on the road to recovery is one of the key reasons that those interested in adding transfer factors to their diets or treatment regimens should do so under the supervision of their physician.

When the body kills off large numbers of infected cells in a short period of time, a toxic reaction, called the Jarisch-Herxheimer reaction, named after the two German dermatologists that characterized it, is to be expected. Those battling deeply embedded infections with stealthy bacteria like Lyme or even problems with yeast overgrowth could be in for a rough ride during the first month or so of transfer factor supplementation, as microbes die and the liver works overtime to clean up toxins spilled into the body.

Regarding the Jarisch-Herxheimer reaction, it is a mistake to presume that feeling ill while undergoing a particular treatment always indicates that one is killing off the pathogen of interest. One might be killing off a different pathogen or experiencing side effects of the treatment. While side effects are uncommon with transfer factors, it is difficult to pin illness experienced during transfer factor therapy on the death of a particular pathogen. The strengthened immune system will go after every pathogen it can find. Further, the increase in levels of inflammatory Th1 cytokines can be uncomfortable on its own.

In short, transfer factors appear to be quite safe. They act by boosting immune system health so that the immune system can attack pathogens. The process of boosting immune system health can lead to mild cold- or flu-like symptoms that seem to resolve early in treatment. In those chronically ill, a die off reaction, called the Jarisch-Herxheimer reaction is always possible. If one is concerned about this, starting slowly is a good idea.

5.4 Where to find them

Until quite recently, transfer factors were only used in hospital settings, most outside of the U.S. They were custom-made for patients from human blood cells in a laboratory and were not available to the public or to most MDs. In the last decade, everything changed. Several companies began using patented processes to extract transfer factors from cow colostrum and chicken eggs. Such extracts are now widely available.

At present, it is quite easy to obtain transfer factors that are broad spectrum, meaning that they are extracted from cow colostrum and/or egg yolks from animals not intentionally exposed to disease causing agents. Broad spectrum transfer factors are extremely powerful immunomodulators that can have a tremendous impact on health, build resistance to infections, help the body fight deep-seated intracellular infections of all kinds, and calm some autoimmune responses and allergies by helping to balance Th1 and Th2 immune activity. Indeed, in the majority of studies discussed in the last chapter, broad spectrum transfer factors were used.

Customized, pathogen-specific transfer factors are harder to find than products containing broad-spectrum transfer factors, but are extremely valuable in the fight against diseases with known pathogens (e.g., Lyme, HIV, herpes viruses, etc). Sources of targeted (pathogen-specific) transfer factors still remain, but must be located through diligent Internet searches or by consulting a knowledgeable physician. Further, some laboratories now offer the service of generating disease-specific transfer factors from a patient's blood samples and will send them to the physician overseeing the patient's care.

A table listing a few of the products currently carried by several companies can be found on the next page. Prices can be obtained from the companies' websites. While some products can be purchased directly by consumers, it is best to use them under the observation of a trained medical practitioner, much the same as any other supplement that affects the health of the body.

It is very important for the reader to be aware that the discussions contained in this book regarding the potential utility of transfer factor supplements for treating and preventing diseases represent the opinions of the author based upon the scientific literature. The views of the author are not necessarily those of the companies that make products containing transfer factors. Further, the author does not endorse particular products containing transfer factors and has no financial ties to the companies making them.

Available products containing transfer factors *

Researched Nutritionals (www.researchednutritionals.com)

Transfer Factor Multi-Immune	Broad spectrum of transfer factors from cow colostrum and chicken eggs, plus a very wide range of ingredients known to boost immune system health (B-12, IP-6, green tea extract, shiitake and maitake mushrooms and others).

4Life Research (www.4life.com)

Transfer Factor Tri-Factor Plus	Broad spectrum of transfer factors from colostrum and chicken eggs, plus nutrients to support immune system health (beta-glucan, maitake and shiitake mushrooms and others).

ProHealth (www.prohealth.com)

Transfer Factor Essentials	Broad spectrum of transfer factors from cow colostrum and chicken eggs, plus a long list of nutrients known to support immune health (beta-glucan, selenium, zinc and others).

Biopharma Scientific (www.biopharmasci.com)

NanoPro PRP	Contains cow colostrum fortified with proline rich polypeptides (transfer factors). Utilizes a proprietary lipid coating that enhances absorption.

ReGen Therapeutics (www.regentherapeutics.com)

Colostrinin	Proline rich polypeptides (transfer factors) from sheep colostrum.

Legacy for Life (www.legacyforlife.net)

i26 Hyperimmune Egg	Powdered egg yolks and egg whites from hens exposed to more than 26 pathogens. Contains all immune fractions, which should include small amounts of transfer factors.

* This is not meant to be an exhaustive list and inclusion of the companies in the table is not an endorsement of either the companies or their products.

5.5 The difference between colostrum supplements and transfer factors

Transfer factors are present in colostrum, the first milk released by female mammals after giving birth. Transfer factors in the colostrum appear to play important roles in programming the offspring's Helper T-cells and stimulating the production of lymphocytes and macrophages. Colostrum can be purchased in supplement form. Why not just take colostrum?

While colostrum can be quite beneficial to health, it contains far more components than a small amount of transfer factors. One must consider whether these extra components will be valuable for a particular condition. According to the Physicians Desk Reference (online at www.PDRhealth.com), cow colostrum contains a great deal of protein and several other components:

> "Other substances found in bovine colostrum include casein, lactoferrin, alpha-lactalbumin, beta-lactoglobulin, and the growth factors insulin-like growth factor-1 (IGF-1), insulin-like growth factor-2 (IGF-2), transforming growth factor beta (TGFbeta) and epidermal growth factor (EGF). In addition, bovine colostrum contains vitamins, minerals, lipids and lactose. Bovine colostrum may also contain colostrinin, also known as proline-rich polypeptide (PRP)"

Note that the terms "colostrinin" and "proline-rich polypeptide" appear to be synonymous with transfer factors.

Once raw colostrum is filtered, the list of components is greatly reduced:

> "Bovine colostrum prepared by microfiltration is mainly composed of whey proteins and their associated immunoglobulins and the growth factors IGF-1, IGF-2, TGFbeta and EGF. Substances such as lactose, fats, casein and lactalbumin are significantly reduced in microfiltered bovine colostrum."

Recall that the gastrointestinal tracts of newborn mammals allow for easier passage of proteins and immunoglobulins (antibodies) into the body. This is not, or should not be, the case in adult mammals. As such, the majority of growth factors and immunoglobulins contained in microfiltered, supplemental colostrum are probably broken down before they get into the body, though some might still get in.

Normally, when a newborn calf feeds on colostrum, microorganisms from the calf go up into a part of the mother's milk sac called the cistern. There, the mother's immune cells crank out antibodies and transfer factors for those particular pathogens. This immune information is then passed back to the calf upon further nursing. The mother produces colostrum for 3-4 days, after which time the calf if switched to bottle feed and the mother is milked.

Colostrum containing pathogen-specific immune information, such as antibodies and transfer factors for Lyme, can be generated by injecting portions of the pathogen into the cistern, where immune cells then respond to it and generate the appropriate immune information to pass back to the calf. Alternatively, it seems that a farmer could just put a tick on the cow and hope it bites! In the end, the colostrum should contain immune information for Lyme and anything else to which the cow has been exposed.

In a fantastic article called "Universal Oral Vaccine – The Immune Milk Saga," Anthony di Fabio from the Arthritis Trust of America explored the use of colostrum in health during the last several decades (di Fabio, 1998). He relayed a fascinating story about a dairy farmer, Herb Saunders, who extracted colostrum from his cows for a Congressman named Berkly Bedell, who had been suffering from Lyme related arthritis. Traditional treatments had failed to improve his condition. Apparently, the Congressman experienced a remarkable recovery as a result of taking colostrum for a few weeks. He testified before Congress about his experience. According to Mr. di Fabio, the testimony played a role in the creation of what is now the National Center for Complementary and Alternative Medicine.

In an unfortunate twist, after the Congressman's testimony, the FDA investigated the dairy farmer. The FDA determined that it only had jurisdiction over state-to-state commerce involving drugs and biological products and could not police the farmer's behavior within his home state. It handed the baton off to the state of Minnesota, which eventually tried Mr. Suanders, twice, unsuccessfully, for practicing medicine without a license. Charges of fraud, swindle and cruelty to animals were dropped before the first trial. Clearly, the patients in this case, Congressmen Bedell and others helped by the colostrum, did not complain. This was purely an issue regarding the legality of using cow colostrum to improve health.

In 2003, the Arthritis Trust of America released a report specifically exploring the legality of using colostrum (ATA, 2003). The report was prepared by Diane Miller, one of the attorneys who represented Mr. Saunders, the dairy farmer mentioned above. It is clear from the article that the laws are complicated. However, the contents of colostrum are food. Ask any newborn infant. It just happens to be food that is rich with information for the immune system. The contents are not drugs, and they are not "biological products," a sort of intermediate between food and drugs.

5.6 Pulsing or daily administration?

Presently, all companies manufacturing products that contain transfer factors recommend daily dosing. The optimal dosing regimen for oral transfer factor supplements remains unclear. Many clinicians have found that pulsing treatments with other immune boosting supplements and drugs, like isoprinosine, is more effective than daily dosing. The concern is that the immune system might learn to ignore a prolonged, steady signal. As such, they recommend pulsing the treatments in some sort of staggered regimen with breaks in between. For instance, rather than daily dosing, as the maker of the isoprinosine-based product Imunovir (Newport Pharmaceuticals) recommends, Dr. Paul Cheney, a ME/CFS specialist, recommends a pattern in which 6 pills are taken per day Monday-Friday during week one, 2 pills per day Monday-Friday during week two. No pills on the weekends. Take every other month off.

While the ideal dosing strategy for transfer factors is not clear, there is no reason to believe that it is *necessary* to take them every day to achieve benefits for immune system health. Indeed, in clinical studies involving injections of transfer factors, administration often follows a weekly or monthly pattern. For these reasons, it is often advisable for those with chronic ailments to begin supplementation with transfer factors very slowly, perhaps once or twice per week, until one knows how their body will react. Just because they *can* be taken daily does not mean that they *must* be taken daily. Some might find that anything beyond a single dose per week evokes too strong an immune response early in treatment. For those with already healthy immune systems, daily dosing seems to be well-tolerated.

In their research on the use of transfer factors for immune-related conditions, the Russian Ministry of Health (2004) used the following dosing strategies for the following conditions. (Note: "TF" and "TF Plus" refer to commercially available products containing transfer factors):

Dosing schedule used in studies by the Russian Ministry of Health (2004)

HIV infection
TF Plus
1 capsule 3 times daily
14 day courses repeated each month

Acute viral hepatitis B
TF
1 capsule 3 times daily
14 day courses repeated each month

Chronic viral hepatitis B and C
TF or TF Plus
1 capsule 3 times daily
14 days each month for the first three months.

Acute Chlamydia
TF Plus and antibiotic
1 capsule 3 times daily
10 days

Psoriasis, atopic dermatitis
TF
1 capsule 3 times daily
14-21 days; repeated courses and during unfavourable seasons of the year

Gastric cancer after surgery
TF Plus
1 capsule 2 times daily
30 days minimal repeated every other month

Duodenal ulcer:

TF Plus

During eradication

2 capsules 3 times daily for 7-10 days

After eradication

1 capsule 3 times daily for the rest of that month

Anti-relapse treatment

1 capsule 2 times daily for 1 month early in spring and late autumn

These dosing strategies were no doubt derived from educated guesses. Also note that broad spectrum, rather than targeted, disease-specific, transfer factor preparations were used. Results were overwhelmingly positive with the broad spectrum formulations. Targeted transfer factors likely would have worked even better.

In short, the optimal pattern for dosing with transfer factors is not known at present. Perhaps the most important piece of information for those with chronic ailments is that it is perfectly fine to start slowly and build up. They do not need to be taken daily, as is clear from studies in which doses were spread out over weeks or months and improvements in health were still observed.

5.7 How long before people who benefit benefit?

Like any other supplement or drug, transfer factors will only be of benefit to those in need of the changes that transfer factors produce. The signals carried by these molecules increase levels of T-cells and Natural Killer cells and help pull the immune system from a Th2 dominated activity profile back toward a balance of Th1 and Th2 responses. Further, transfer factors raised against specific pathogens can help orient the immune response toward those pathogens.

For those who benefit from these changes, the length of time between the first capsule and improved health is unpredictable. Further, symptoms can be exacerbated on the way to improvement.

Dr. Carol Ann Ryser, MD — the Medical Director of Health Centers of America — has been using transfer factor supplements in her practice since 1998. In 2001, she was interviewed by a company, ProHealth, that carries products containing transfer factors. In addition to selling supplements, ProHealth serves as a vast clearinghouse for information on immune-related conditions. Indeed, the company's founder, Rich Carson, has suffered from ME/CFS for well over two decades. Here is a snippet of the interview with Dr. Ryser. (See "Stiff" in the reference list for a link to the full transcript.)

> **ImmuneSupport.com**: "How long does it usually take for a patient to experience positive results once they start taking transfer factor?"

> **Dr. Ryser**: "My patients usually start to feel better within 3-6 months of beginning treatment with transfer factor. Dramatic results usually manifest in about one year, but we really begin to see positive changes in 5-6 months. It typically takes about a year of transfer factor treatment to really turn a patient around. I am specifically referring to chronically ill patients who have an average of 2-7 chronic infections that require treatment. The body's cells regenerate every six months, and you need to give the body a chance to generate healthy cells before dramatic improvements in a patient's overall health can emerge."

Dr. Ryser indicated that she has seen tremendous improvements in health for those with chronic viral infections, even for extremely ill patients. However, many relapse if they make the decision to stop taking them once their health improves, thus requiring regular use, perhaps throughout life. Such relapses suggest that some of the patients she refers to suffer from an underlying immune imbalance, and that this imbalance renders the individuals susceptible to infections, thus requiring continual treatment to keep the immune system on point. It is entirely unknown how long treatment should persist in those suffering from discrete infections that respond positively to transfer factor therapy. In any case, a commitment to taking a daily, oral supplement to help the body stay one step ahead of an illness seems like a fair trade, particularly in situations where one's health is poor without treatment.

Taking transfer factors under the observation of a physician allows for more objective measures of improvements. For instance, for those with low Natural Killer cell levels and high levels of peptides in the complement cascade (e.g., C3a and C4a) at baseline, levels can be tracked to assess whether improvements in subjective states can be correlated with objective lab results. The same is true for those showing high levels of autoimmune-related antibodies, such as rheumatoid factor in rheumatoid arthritis and TPOAb in autoimmune thyroid disease. While not necessary, having such lab analyses conducted while taking transfer factors can help ensure that recovery is on track and that transfer factors are contributing to it.

5.8 Summary

In summary, transfer factors are small molecules generated by Helper T-cells. They can boost immune health and potentially help the human body deal with diseases. In supplement form, transfer factors are currently protected by the

Dietary Supplement Health and Education Act of 1994 here in the U.S. There are no guarantees that they will impact a person's health. However, based upon the science, they should at least be considered if you, or even your household pets, have been ill with conditions related to the immune system. There are also reasons to expect that daily, supplemental use of transfer factors should improve immune system status even in already healthy people.

Before deciding to incorporate products containing transfer factors into your daily regimen of supplements, please discuss this possibility with your physician. Be forewarned that most MDs will likely dismiss the idea of transfer factors when first raised. Despite the utility of transfer factors in treating and preventing diseases, few MDs have thus far become aware of them. Providing your physician with this text, including the scientific abstracts in Appendix I, can help catch them up to speed so that they can advise you on the correct course of action.

Chapter 6

What roles might transfer factors play in the future of medicine?

Transfer factors have powerful effects on immune system function, particularly on cells and chemical messengers utilized in the cell-mediated (Th1) immune pathway – the pathway that allows the body to identify and destroy infected self cells and cancer cells. Research suggests that transfer factors are effective at helping the immune system deal with a variety of infections and conditions, including tuberculosis, streptococcus, HIV, CMV, Epstein-Barr, HHV-6, arthritis, Candida, ME/CFS, and the herpes viruses that cause cold sores, genital outbreaks and shingles. Several published scientific studies also suggest that transfer factors hold promise in preventing infections before they occur by conveying immunity to specific pathogens.

Unlike pharmaceutical drugs, transfer factors act by helping the immune system do its job. Transfer factors are a natural component of the strategy used by the body to protect itself against disease. Transfer factors bind to antigens on infected self cells and target these cells for destruction. By communicating information to the immune system in a language it understands inherently, supplemental transfer factors strengthen the cell-mediated immune response and increase the number of Natural Killer cells and Cytotoxic T-cells available for destroying non-self cells, infected self cells and cancer cells. Transfer factors safely and effectively help the body locate and destroy stubborn viral and bacterial infections and rebalance the immune dysfunction associated with many disease states.

Transfer factors offer a promising new approach for battling infectious diseases and cancers. Given what is known about the utility of transfer factors at present, what might the future hold for transfer factors in the treatment and prevention of diseases?

6.1 Future uses of transfer factors

Transfer factors could help fill large gaps in disease treatment and prevention left open by our over-reliance on antibiotics, vaccines, antivirals and immunosuppressants. Pending more science, transfer factors could become first line treatments – and means of prevention – for diseases like:

- HIV
- HPV
- Lyme
- Herpes viruses
- Measles, mumps and rubella
- Cold
- Flu (H1N1 and H5N1)
- Candida
- Tuberculosis

(cont'd)

- SARS
- West Nile virus
- Norovirus
- H. pylori
- Hepatitis A, B, C,* D and E
- Bartonella
- Cancers
- XMRV

...and a long list of others

More than 1000 papers have been published on the subject of transfer factors, earning them a place in medicine. They cannot replace all medications used to fight disease. However, their unique mechanisms of action and safety profile allow them to be used along with many existing options. Let us explore how transfer factors could be used alongside two of the primary tools used currently to fight disease – antibiotics and vaccines – as we move further into the 21st century.

---

*Note: Hepatitis C (HCV) is the leading cause of liver transplant in the US and 100,000+ new cases are reported annually. At present, treatments are limited to cytokines and antivirals with serious side effects. This is an *ideal* virus against which to assess the public health benefits of transfer factors. Those given HCV specific transfer factors should show rapid improvements in liver enzyme profiles. Fewer acute infections should become chronic and the number of new cases in those at risk should go down.

6.2 Transfer factors in the era of antibiotic-resistant bacteria

When penicillin became widely available in the 1940s and 50s, the relationship between humans and bacteria suddenly changed in profound ways. With ease, penicillin cleared up bacterial infections, like staph infections, that normally would have killed a person. The effectiveness of penicillin against bacteria must have led many to believe that the days of danger-ous bacterial infections were over. Such elation would have been short-lived, however. Within a few years of the dawn of wide-spread use of antibiotics, it became clear that penicillin-resistant strains of bacteria were emerging. In the 50 or so years since, there has been an ongoing race between researchers developing new antibiotics and bacteria developing resistance to them. So far, but perhaps not for much longer, researchers have been leading by a nose.

Antibiotic resistance in bacteria spreads in two directions – *vertically* and *horizontally*. In the case of vertical spread, those bacteria that have become resistant to one or several types of antibiotics pass those genes on when they divide and create new cells, sort of like passing on genetic material to offspring. Horizontal spread of resistance occurs when non-resistant bacteria acquire resistance from other bacteria that already have it. Given current concerns about antibiotic resistance, it is worth taking a look at some examples of these two types of spread in more detail. We will then discuss how transfer factors can help pick up the slack created by failing antibiotics.

As with all other organisms that undergo cell division, when bacteria divide, there is a chance that the genetic material in the DNA will not be copied perfectly. These errors in copy-ing, or mutations, can lead to changes in the cell's form and/or function. Typically, such errors hurt bacteria rather than help. However, every now and then, they hit the jackpot and the phenotypic (observable) changes emerging from those errors in gene copying allow the bacteria to avoid succumbing to antibio-tics. For example, penicillin kills bacteria by sticking to an enzyme that helps create the cell wall. With penicillin stuck to it, the enzyme does not work, the cell wall cannot be maintained, and the bacteria die. A genetic mutation that creates a functional enzyme to which penicillin does not stick renders the penicillin useless. Alternatively, the bacteria could create way too much of the enzyme to which penicillin binds so that the penicillin cannot disable all of them, or the bacteria might begin creating an enzyme that actually dismantles the penicillin molecule. Once such mutations occur, they are passed on through the DNA during subsequent cell division, leading to vertical spread of resistance.

Bacteria can also acquire resistance from other bacteria that have it. This can happen in several ways. In a process called *conjugative transposition*, bacteria swap bits of genetic material with each other. This is one of the more frightening processes leading to resistance, because only one type of bacteria needs to develop resistance in order to begin spreading resistance to unrelated species. This is one of the primary ways that resistance develops in bacteria that commonly cause infections in hospitals.

Bacteria can also pick up bits of free-floating DNA from the remnants of dead bacteria. If they are lucky, these fragments convey resistance to antibiotics. In both cases – conjugative transposition and picking up free-floating DNA – resistance can be acquired by a species of bacteria rather than developed by it. Once acquired via horizontal spread, the resistance is passed down through vertical spread.

Overuse of antibiotics in humans, failure to complete full courses of antibiotic treatment, and widespread administration of antibiotics to livestock (in the hopes of promoting growth, not treating infections) increase the odds that bacteria will evolve resistance to antibiotics. By continually exposing bacteria to our arsenal of weapons against them, we give them the opportunity to develop ways around them. The more we use the weapons, the greater likelihood that resistance to them will emerge.

At present, we still have an edge over bacteria, but only a slight one. The situation is not quite as dire as many think, but it is not good. Since the dawn of mass production of penicillin, over 10 distinct classes of antibiotics have been discovered, with dozens upon dozens of different varieties within those classes. Unfortunately, bacteria have developed resistance to drugs in every class. Vancomycin, approved by the FDA in 1958, has long been considered a weapon of last resort. Bacteria have proven that vancomycin, too, is beatable. Concern over this development is captured in the following passage from a 1995 article published by the FDA (Lewis, 1995):

> "Vancomycin-resistant enterococci were first reported in England and France in 1987, and appeared in one New York City hospital in 1989. By 1991, 38 hospitals in the United States reported the bug. By 1993, 14 percent of patients with enterococcus in intensive-care units in some hospitals had vancomycin-resistant strains, a 20-fold increase from 1987. A frightening report came in 1992, when a British researcher observed a transfer of a vancomycin-resistant gene from enterococcus to Staph aureus in the laboratory. Alarmed, the researcher immediately destroyed the bacteria."

Fortunately, new drugs are on the horizon and should keep us in the race for a while. In 2005, researchers from a biotech company in Denmark published a manuscript in the journal *Nature* in which they report isolating a class of antimicrobials, called defensins, from fungi. A variety of cells in the human body, including cells lining the intestines, produce defensins to ward off pathogens looking for cells to infect, so defensins from fungi could prove quite useful. Further, in early 2009, research funded by Pfizer, and published in the *Proceedings of the National Academy of Sciences*, yielded a unique class of antibiotics based on molecules (pyridopyrimidines) that block fat synthesis in bacteria. Let us hope these new discoveries move from the bench-top to the medicine-shop soon!

Transfer factors hold tremendous promise in helping the body defeat chronic bacterial infections, including chronic Lyme, tuberculosis, Bartonella, Erlichia, chlamydia pneumonia and others, even in cases where long-term antibiotic treatment fails. Both intracellular and extracellular bacteria are destroyed by the types of cells spurred into action by transfer factors. Because transfer factors act through the immune system and do not attack pathogens directly, they cannot replace antibiotics as first line treatments for acute bacterial infections, but should be useful as supportive treatment in such cases due to their immune enhancing effects.

6.3 Transfer factors and traditional vaccines

In addition to helping patients beat diseases they have already contracted, transfer factors could be used in ways similar to traditional vaccines, protecting people against diseases before they have been exposed to them. Indeed, that is how they were initially discovered by Dr. Lawrence in the 1940s.

Researchers in China speculate that transfer factors will be useful in preventing hepatitis B (Xu YP et al, 2006). Researchers in Italy recently made a similar argument for the use of transfer factors in preventing newly emerging strains of bird flu (Pizza et al, 2006). Transfer factors could be used to help prevent infections with dozens of other pathogens, as well.

The Human Papilloma Virus (HPV) is a virus that can be transmitted sexually and is thought to be the causative agent behind many cases of cervical cancer – up to 70%. Cervical cancer is curable if caught early and afflicts around 15,000 women per year. For comparison, breast cancer strikes somewhere near 200,000 women. A vaccine for HPV has been approved by the FDA and is recommended for girls aged 11 or 12. It requires three injections during six months, and is considered safe, though reports of possible side effects are now surfacing. Transfer factors can be made easily for HPV. In fact, they already have been.

It would be of interest to determine whether oral transfer factors for HPV could replace the injectable vaccine. It would be an important step for public health, but might not go over well with drug companies, like Merck, which makes the HPV vaccine, Gardasil. For Gardisil, the cost per vaccination is $360. In 2007, Texas teetered on becoming the first state to require HPV vaccination for all school aged girls. Other states also have considered such a measure. Vaccination for HPV is becoming quite popular in European countries, as well, suddenly making the HPV vaccine market a very lucrative one. Despite widespread reports of side effects associated with Gardasil and other HPV vaccines, their use continues to rise.

There are several advantages to the use of transfer factors for immunization relative to the use of vaccines. Kirkpatrick and Rozzo (1995), in their patent application for generating purified antigen-specific transfer factors, summarize some of these advantages as follows:

> "The advantages of using transfer factors to impart immunity are many. They include speed of transfer of immunity. Immunity to a specific antigen can be detected in as little as several hours after administration of the transfer factor...The recipients acquire specific immunity in 24 to 48 hours. This is much more rapid than the 2 to 6 weeks required for induction of immunity by conventional vaccines.
>
> Because each unique transfer factor molecule is thought to transfer immunity to a specific antigen or epitope, several different transfer factor molecules specific for different antigens can be ad-

mixed to custom design a complex immune response.

The substantially pure transfer factor allows one to determine the amino acid sequence of a particular transfer factor and, given this information, one can synthesize the transfer factor either chemically or by recombinant methods. Thus, as a result of the present invention, large quantities of transfer factor can now be produced. This will allow transfer of a desired immune response to large numbers of humans or animals.

In addition, the storage of transfer factor is another advantage. Transfer factor molecules that are contemplated as part of the present invention are very stable. Thus, according to the present invention, the transfer factor molecules do not require extraordinary precaution to maintain or administer the material."

While both transfer factors and vaccines can be used to impart immunity, transfer factors can be made more quickly, in larger quantities, transported without special precautions, taken orally and have fewer side effects. Whether transfer factors are as effective as vaccines in conveying immunity to a disease in a large population is left to be determined. Given the proven effectiveness of vaccines for many infectious agents, perhaps a combination of transfer factors and vaccines would be ideal in many cases. For those infectious agents difficult to fight with vaccines, transfer factors could be studied for use as monotherapy.

6.4 Transfer factors and next-generation vaccines

In early 2009, researchers at the Dana-Farber Cancer Institute in Boston, Massachusetts, the Burnham Institute for Medical Research in La Jolla, California, the Centers for Disease Control and the National Institute on Allergies and Infectious Diseases, announced a major breakthrough in medicine that should lead to superior replacements for many old-style vaccines.

The researchers discovered that viruses, flu viruses in this case, contain a clump of protein that mutates quickly. It is this clump of protein to which most antibodies for flu attach, making it nearly impossible for the body to keep up with the rate of mutation and thereby prevent re-infection. More importantly, they discovered areas just beneath that protein clump that do not change as much and are shared across multiple strains of flu. Antibodies made against these regions of the virus are smaller in number, but much more effective at preventing re-infection with flu. Indeed, once bound to the virus, these antibodies prevent the virus from changing shape, thus denying the virus the ability to enter into healthy cells.

By extracting such antibodies and administering them to patients, these antibodies could be used to convey immunity to flu in much the same way that transfer factors are used. While considered an advance in the domain of vaccine research, this approach is more like the use of transfer factors than vaccines. Both involve the use of pathogen-specific peptides made in the body. The combination of transfer factors for flu (or other viruses) and antibodies for flu (or other viruses) could prove incredibly valuable for public health and disease prevention. The antibodies would tag the virus early on and transfer factors would help prevent intracellular infections.

6.5 If transfer factors have so much potential in medicine, why does the medical community seem so unaware of them?

More than 1000 manuscripts about transfer factors have been published in the past 50 years and can be located through the U.S. National Library of Medicine's search engine, Med-Line/PubMed (www.pubmed.gov). Despite decades of research and compelling findings, most medical practitioners seem unaware of transfer factors.

In general, the disconnect between current dogma in medicine and the actual state of medical science is perhaps best explained by a 2003 article in the *New England Journal of Medicine*, which suggests that most practicing MDs are 10-20 years behind in the literature and make decisions based on antiquated training.

Perhaps because of false confidence in current approaches for disease management, misplaced trust in the pharmaceutical industry, the difficulties many MDs have in keeping up with the scientific literature, the lack of concern over most viral infections and the pervasive belief that chronic bacterial infections are rare, transfer factors have flown under the radar, at least in the U.S. Transfer factors have been studied extensively outside of the U.S. In 2004, based on their own clinical studies, the Russian Ministry of Health endorsed transfer factors as first line treatments for a variety of immune conditions.

The current situation regarding the reluctance of physicians to embrace the use of transfer factors, and the hope that the situation will change, is nicely captured by Viza (1996). Despite the fact that more than 10 years have passed since the publication of the article, the comments remain valid.

"In the realm of inductive science, the dominant paradigm can seldom be challenged in a frontal attack, especially when it is apparently successful, and only what Kuhn calls 'scientific revolutions' can overthrow it. Thus, it is hardly surprising that the concept of transfer factor is considered with contempt, and the existence of the moiety improbable… [However] because of the failure of medical science to manage the AIDS pandemic, transfer factor, which has been successfully used for treating or preventing viral infections, may today overcome a priori prejudice and rejection more swiftly."

Medical dogma is slow to change. Let us hope that a paradigm shift comes soon in this case!

6.6 The value of transfer factors for healthy people

Transfer factors appear to be quite safe, at least for those subjects included in clinical studies thus far, and have known efficacy against a wide range of pathogens. Transfer factors are powerful immunomodulators and trigger increases in levels of Natural Killer cells, Helper T-cells, Cytotoxic T-cells, macrophages and others. All of these cells are important for protecting the body from disease. Given the immune boosting affects of transfer factors, an individual need not be ill to benefit from their use.

Americans spend more than $20 billion every year on supplements. Anyone who routinely takes supplements in an effort to indirectly boost immune system activity would likely benefit more from transfer factors than from common supplements like zinc, Echinacea, and various vitamins. Boosting the immune system not only improves current health, it can help stave off future infections. According to a Cornell University publication, "Top 10 Health Topics: Cold, Flu and Strep Throat":

"Everything you can do to maintain a healthy immune system will bolster your chances of reducing the severity of an illness or avoiding it altogether."

The literature is clear that transfer factors boost immune system health in a variety of ways. As such, they should have great utility for healthy people interested in maintaining an immune system capable of protecting them from common ailments like cold and flu, from cancerous cells, and from re-emerging pathogens like those that cause herpes outbreaks, tuberculosis and even polio.

6.6 All systems check

This book focuses on the immune system and the role of transfer factors in its operation. It is beyond the scope of the book to explore in great detail how the immune system interacts with other systems in the body. However, as savvy readers are certainly aware, the immune system does not function in isolation. Indeed, in many cases of immune dysfunction, the root cause resides elsewhere. Problems in the pituitary, the master gland that regulates hormone levels in the thyroid and adrenals. Mitochondrial dysfunction leading to energy starvation throughout all of the systems. Chronic activation of the sympathetic (fight or flight) branch of the nervous system, sometimes in a desperate attempt to keep the body going. Often all of the above at the same time and more.

Understanding, detecting and treating diseases requires a multi-systems approach. Rational as that might seem, the current medical system precludes taking a pragmatic approach and favors a one doctor for one organ system mentality. As such, a patient with a chronic condition that involves the heart, lungs and brain, and includes symptoms of pain, depression and fatigue, might see a dozen different MDs, have a dozen different diagnoses and be treated for each problem separately. Without communication between these various specialists, and no one searching for the underlying source of all of the problems, the patient has little hope of truly recovering.

It is a common logical mistake to focus too intently on one aspect of physiology when trying to treat and defeat a disease. Huge gains in health can result from addressing specific aspects of dysfunction, like cholesterol, blood pressure, or thyroid hormone levels. However, it is usually when denominators common to multiple symptoms are identified and addressed that health improves in leaps and bounds. As science continues to reveal the inner workings of the human machine, the ability to discern and correct the underlying causes of diseases should improve. Until then, finding a physician capable of exploring all of the systems in the body at once can be quite helpful, though rare at the moment and almost always out-of-network in the U.S. with regard to insurance coverage.

Ultimately, health is a state of dynamic harmony, or allostasis, within the body. With regard to the immune system, transfer factors have proven themselves quite valuable for helping to re-establish balance.

6.7 Review and discussion

Transfer factors are small molecules generated by the immune system. They are used by immune cells to communicate with, and coordinate the activity of, other immune cells throughout the body. They are not species-specific, meaning that transfer factors generated by cows, chickens, and other animals can augment immune system activity in any other species – including humans and household pets (they were used in veterinary medicine before becoming available for human consumption.)

Clinical and scientific research, reviewed in previous chapters, strongly suggests that transfer factors are capable of boosting human immune system health on a grand scale. For healthy people, this can make them even healthier. For ill people, this could improve the quality of their lives.

Improving immune system health is an understudied approach to dealing with many diseases, in part because advances in the diagnosis and treatment of diseases have become intimately – too intimately – tied to drug development by pharmaceutical companies.

Transfer factors are not drugs. They carry information that, when read by immune cells, can cause the immune system to become more active and vigilant. Transfer factors, whether purified or in colostrum, are nature's answer to viral, mycobacterial and CWD-bacterial infections. Transfer factors derived from cow colostrum and egg yolks are protected as supplements under law.

Transfer factors carry minimal risks of side effects, with the exception of mild flu-like symptoms that generally occur sometime during the first few weeks of taking them. These symptoms are temporary and are viewed as evidence that the immune system has been activated and is on the hunt for intracellular infections. Those who have been ill for quite some time, and who respond positively to transfer factors, should expect an exacerbation of symptoms on the way to healing. This is normal and is one of the factors that should be carefully considered before deciding whether to take them.

Regardless of their safety profile, as is the case with anything else that comes in a capsule, it is very important to make careful, informed decisions before taking them. Any substance that impacts how the body functions could have undesirable effects. It is impossible to know how each individual will react to something like transfer factors, so please inform your doctor if you intend to take them. Chances are good that your doctor is unaware that transfer factors exist or are available. Titles and abstracts of 160 studies conducted on transfer factors over the past 60 years are included in Appendix 1 for the purpose of helping your doctor get caught up to speed. The detailed review of the scientific literature contained in this book should also be of benefit for them.

It is the author's sincere hope that this book has been of use and that the material has helped readers make sense of their immune systems and perhaps the pathologies that plague them. There are options for improving health that do not require drug companies, prescriptions or injections. Transfer factors represent one such option.

Best of luck with your health!

References

Ablashi DV, Eastman HB, Owen CB, Roman MM, Friedman J, Zabriskie JB, Peterson DL, Pearson GR, Whitman JE. Frequent HHV-6 reactivation in multiple sclerosis (MS) and chronic fatigue syndrome (CFS) patients. J Clin Virol. 2000 May;16(3):179-91.

Ablashi DV, Levine PH, DeVinci C et al Use of anti HHV-6 transfer factor for the treatment of two patients with chronic fatigue syndrome (CFS). Two case reports. Biotherapy 1996;9:81-86.

AHA. Inflammation, heart disease and stroke: The role of C reactive protein. Ameican Heart Association. 2007. (accessed online August 8, 2007 at: http://www.americanheart.org/presenter.jhtml?identifie r=4648)

Amsterdam JD, Maislin G, Rybakowski J. A possible antiviral action of lithium carbonate in herpes simplex virus infections. Biological Psychiatry 1990;27(4):447-453.

Arnon R, Aharoni R. Mechanisms of action of glatiramer acetate in multiple sclerosis and its potential for the development of new applications. Proc Natl Acad Sci. 2004;5:14593-14598.

ATA. Colostrum therapy legal evaluation. 2003. The Arthritis Trust of America (available online: http://www.arthritistrust.org/articclesmisc.htm)

Balfour A. The infective granule in certain protozoal infections, as illustrated by the spirochaetosis of Sudanese fowl. British Medical Journal. 1911;1:752.

Basten A, McLeod JG, Pollard JD, Walsh JC, Stewart GJ, Garrick R, Frith JA, Van Der Brink CM.Transfer factor in treatment of multiple sclerosis. Lancet. 1980 1;2(8201):931-4.

Behan PO. Durward WF. Melville ID. McGeorge AP. Behan WM. Transfer-factor therapy in multiple sclerosis. Lancet. 1976;1(7967):988-90.

Benlahrech A, Harris J, Meiser A et al. Adenovirus vector vaccination induces expansion of memory CD4 T cells with mucosal homing phenotype that are readily susceptible to HIV-1. PNAS. 2009;106:19940-19945.

Bennett MP, Zeller JM, Rosenberg L, McCann J. The effect of mirthful laughter on stress and natural killer cell activity. Altern Ther Health Med. 2003;9(2):38-45.

Beran B, Havelkova M, Kaustova J, Dvorska L, Pavlik I. Cell wall deficient forms of mycobacteria: a review. Veterinarni Medicina. 2006;51(7):365-389.

Bilikiewicz A, Gaus W. Colostrinin (a naturally occurring, proline-rich, polypeptide mixture) in the treatment of Alzheimer's disease. J Alzheimers Dis. 2004;6(1):17-26.

Bock SJ. Transfer factor and its clinical applications. International Journal of Integrative Medicine. 2000; 2(4):44-49.

Bock K, Bock S. 12 strategies to support your immune system, Part 3. Posted and retrieved October 12, 2007, from http://rhinebeckhealth.blogspot.com/2007/10/12-strategies-to-support-your-immune.html

Burgdorfer W. Keynote Address - The Complexity of Vector-borne Spirochetes. 12th International Conference on Lyme Disease and Other Spirochetal and Tick-Borne Disorders. New York City, April 9-10, 1999. (Accessed online January 11, 2009 at: http://www.medscape.com/viewarticle/429454)

Burrascano JJ. Diagnostic hints and treatment guidelines for Lyme and other tick borne illnesses. 14th Ed. ILADS 2002 (online at: www.ilads.org/burrascano_1102.html)

Cantorna MT. Vitamin D and its role in immunology: multiple sclerosis, and inflammatory bowel disease. Prog Biophys Mol Biol. 2006;92(1):60-4.

Carey JT, Lederman MM, Toossi Z, Edmonds K, Hodder S, Calabrese LH, Proffitt MR, Johnson CE, Ellner JJ. Augmentation of skin test reactivity and lymphocyte blastogenesis in patients with AIDS treated with transfer factor. JAMA. 1987;257(5):651-5.

CDC. Nonpharmaceutical interventions for pandemic influenza, international measures. Emerging Infectious Diseases 2006; 12(1), 81-87.

Cohly HH. Panja A. Immunological findings in autism. International Review of Neurobiology. 2005;71:317-41.

Cruess DG, Antoni MH, Gonzalez J, Fletcher MA, Klimas N, Duran R, Ironson G, Schneiderman N. Sleep disturbance mediates the association between psychological distress and immune status among HIV-positive men and women on combination antiretroviral therapy. J Psychosom Res. 2003;54(3):185-9.

Dantzer R, Kelley KW. Twenty years of research on cytokine-induced sickness behavior. Brain Behav Immun. 2006 Nov 4 ahead of print

de Andres C, Aristimuno C, de Las Heras V, Martinez-Gines ML, Bartolome M, Arroyo R, Navarro J, Gimenez-Roldan S, Fernandez-Cruz E, Sanchez-Ramon S. Interferon beta-1a therapy enhances CD4+ regulatory T-cell function: an ex vivo and in vitro longitudinal study in relapsing-remitting multiple sclerosis. J Neuroimmunol. 2007;182(1-2):204-11.

De Vinci C. Levine PH. Pizza G. Fudenberg HH. Orens P. Pearson G. Viza D. Lessons from a pilot study of transfer factor in chronic fatigue syndrome. Biotherapy. 1996;9(1-3):87-90.

di Fabio A. Universal oral vaccine – The immune milk saga. 1998. The Arthritis Trust of America. (available online: http://www.arthritistrust.org/articclesmisc.htm)

Diamond M, Kelly JP, Connor TJ. Antidepressants suppress production of the Th1 cytokine interferon-gamma, independent of monoamine transporter blockade. European Neuropsychopharmacology 2006;16:481-490.

Eastman CI, Young MA, Fogg LF, Liu L, Meaden PM. Bright light treatment of winter depression: a placebo-controlled trialArch Gen Psychiatry. 1998;55(10):883-9.

Estrada-Parra S, Nagaya A, Serrano E, Rodriguez O, Santamaria V, Ondarza R, Chavez R, Correa B, Monges A, Cabezas R, Calva C, Estrada-Garcia I. Comparative study of transfer factor and acyclovir in the treatment of herpes zoster. Int J Immunopharmacol. 1998;20(10):521-35.

Estrada-Parra S, Chavez-Sanchez R, Ondarza-Aguilera R, Correa-Meza B, Serrano-Miranda E, Monges-Nicolau A, Calva-Pellicer C. Immunotherapy with transfer factor of recurrent herpes simplex type I. Arch Med Res. 1995;26 Spec No:S87-92.

Faber WR, Leiker DL, Nengerman IM, Schellekens PT. A placebo controlled clinical trial of transfer factor in lepromatous leprosy. Clin Exp Immunol. 1979 ;35(1):45-52.

Fabre RA, Perez TM, Aguilar LD, Rangel MJ, Estrada-Garcia I, Hernandez-Pando R, Estrada Parra S. Transfer Factors as immunotherapy and supplement of chemotherapy in experimental pulmonary tuberculosis. Clin Exp Immunol. 2004;136(2):215-23.

Fan H. A new human retrovirus associated with prostate cancer. PNAS. 2007;104(5):1449-1450

Fernandez-Ortega C, Dubed M, Ramos Y, Navea L, Alvarez G. Lobaina L, Lopez L, Casillas D, Rodriguez L. Non-induced leukocyte extract reduces HIV replication and TNF secretion. Biochemical & Biophysical Research Communications. 2004;325(3):1075-81.

Fidel PL, Lynch ME, Sobel JD. Candida-specific cell-mediated immunity is demonstrable in mice with experimental vaginal candidiasis. Infect Immunity. 1993;61:1990–1995.

Franco-Molina MA, Mendoza-Gamboa E, Miranda-Hernández D, Zapata-Benavides P, Castillo-León L, Isaza-Brando C, Tamez-Guerra Rs, Rodríguez-Padilla C. In vitro effects of bovine dialyzable leukocyte extract (bDLE) in cancer cells. Cytotherapy. 2006;8:408-414.

Franco-Molina MA, Mendoza-Gamboa E, Zapata-Benavides P, Vera-García ME, Castillo-Tello P, García de la Fuente A, Mendoza RD, Garza RG, Támez-Guerra RS, Rodríguez-Padilla C. ImmunePotent CRP (bovine dialyzable leukocyte extract) adjuvant immunotherapy: a phase I study in non-small cell lung cancer patients. Cytotherapy 2008;10(5):490-6.

Frith JA, McLeod JG, Basten A, Pollard JD, Hammond SR, Williams DB. Crossie PA.Transfer factor as a therapy for multiple sclerosis: a follow-up study. Clinical & Experimental Neurology. 1986;22:149-54.

Gaudreault E, Gosselin J. Leukotriene B4 induces release of antimicrobial peptides in the lungs of virally infected mice. J Immunology. 2008;180:6211-6221.

Georgescu C. Effect of long-term therapy with transfer factor in rheumatoid arthritis. Med Interne. 1985;23(2):135-40.

Gorman C, Park A, Thompson D. Salk vaccine for AIDS. Time. February 6, 1995. (Accessed online January 10, 2009 at http://www.time.com/time/magazine/article/0,9171,98 2431-2,00.html

Granitov VM, Karbysheva NV, Sultanov LV, McCausland C, Oganova E. Usage of Transfer Factor Plus in Treatment of HIV - Infected Patients. Russian Journal of HIV, AIDS and Related Problems. 2002;1:79-80.

Grohn P. Anttila R. Krohn K. The effect of non-specifically acting transfer factor component on cellular immunity in juvenile rheumatoid arthritis. Scandinavian Journal of Rheumatology. 1976;5(3):151-7.

Haber MJ et al Effectiveness of interventions to reduce contact rates during a simulated influenza pandemic. Emerging Infectious Diseases. 2007;13(4):581-589.

Heller IR. Starvation Diet: FDA Lacks Adequate Resources for its Nutritional Health and Consumer Protection Missions. Center for Science in the Public Interest. 2003. (Available at: www.cspinet.org)

Hennen WJ, Lisonbee DT. U.S. Patent 6,468,534 B1, 2002.

Holick MF.Vitamin D: its role in cancer prevention and treatment. Prog Biophys Mol Biol. 2006 ;92(1):49-59.

Holman AJ, Myers RR. A randomized, double-blind, placebo-controlled trial of pramipexole, a dopamine agonist, in patients with fibromyalgia receiving concomitant medications. Arthritis Rheum. 2005;52:2495-505.

Homann D. Teyton L. Oldstone MBA. Differential regulation of antiviral T-cell immunity results in stable CD8+ but declining CD4+ T-cell memory. Nature Med. 2001;7:913-919.

Hoyeraal HM. Froland SS. Salvesen CF. Munthe E. Natvig JB. Kass E. Blichfeldt P. Hegna TM. Revlem E. Sandstad B. Hjort NL. No effect of transfer factor in juvenile rheumatoid arthritis by double-blind trial. Annals of the Rheumatic Diseases. 1978;37(2):175-9.

Hughes RA. Immunological treatment of multiple sclerosis. J Neurol. 1983;230(2):73-80.

Hyun KJ, Kondo M, Koh T, Tokura H, Tamotsu S, Oishi T.Effect of dim and bright light exposure on some immunological parameters measured under thermal neutral conditions. Chronobiol Int. 2005;22(6):1145-55.

Iushkova TA, Iushkov VV. The immunomodulating activity of a transfer-factor preparation transflavin, specific to tick-borne encephalitis virus. Zh Mikrobiol Epidemiol Immunobiol. 1998 Mar-Apr;(2):83-5.

Janeway CA, Travers P, Walport M, Shlomchik MJ. *Immunobiology : The immune system in health and disease, 5th Ed.* New

York: Garland Publishing. 2001. (accessed online at: http://www.ncbi.nlm.nih.gov/books/bv.fcgi?rid=imm)

Jones JF, Jeter WS, Fulginiti VA et al Treatment of childhood combined Epstein-Barr virus/cytomegalovirus infection with oral bovine transfer factor. Lancet 1981;2:122-124.

Khan A. Hansen B. Hill NO. Loeb E. Pardue AS. Hill JM. Transfer factor in the treatment of herpes simplex types 1 and 2. Dermatologica. 163(2):177-85, 1981

Kass E, Froland SS, Natvig JB, Blichfeldt P, Hoyeraal HM. Letter: Transfer factor in juvenile rheumatoid arthritis. Lancet. 1974;1(7858):627-8.

Katoch K. Immunotherapy of leprosy. Indian J Lepr. 1996;68(4):349-61.

Ketchel SJ, Rodriguez V, Stone A, Gutterman JU. A study of transfer factor for opportunistic infections in cancer patients. Medical & Pediatric Oncology. 1979;6(4):295-301.

Kidd P. Th1/Th2 balance: The hypothesis, its limitations, and implications for health and disease. Altern Med Rev. 2003;8(3):223-46.

Kidd PM. Autism, an extreme challenge to integrative medicine. Part 2: medical management. Altern Med Rev. 2002;7(6):472-99.

Kimball JW. *Vaccines*. (Accessed January 10, 2009 at http://biology-pages.info)

Kirkpatrick CH. Transfer Factors: identification of conserved sequences in transfer factor molecules. Mol Med. 2000;6(4):332-41.

Kirkpatrick CH. Activities and characteristics of Transfer Factors. Biotherapy. 1996;9(1-3):13-6.

Kirkpatrick CH. Structural nature and functions of Transfer Factors. Ann N Y Acad Sci. 1993;23:362-8.

Kirkpatrick CH. Biological response modifiers. Interferons, interleukins, and transfer factor. Ann Allergy. 1989;62(3):170-6.

Kirkpatrick CH, Rozzo SJ. Transfer factors and methods of use. U.S. Patent 5470835, filed July 22, 1994, and issued November 28, 1995.

Kogelnik AM, Loomis K, Hoegh-Petersen M, Rosso F, Hischier C, Montoya JG. Use of valganciclovir in patients with elevated antibody titers against Human Herpesvirus-6 (HHV-6) and Epstein-Barr Virus (EBV) who were experiencing central nervous system dysfunction including long-standing fatigue. J Clin Virol. 2006; 37 Suppl 1: S33-8.

Kruzel ML, Janusz M, Lisowski J, Fischleigh RV, Georgiades JA. Towards an understanding of biological role of colostrinin peptides. J Mol Neurosci. 2001;17(3):379-89.

Lang I, Nekam H, Gergely P et al Effect of in vivo and in vitro treatment with Dialyzable Leukocyte Extract on human natural killer cell activity. Clin Immunol and Immunopathol 1982;25:139-144.

Lawrence HS, Borkowsky W. Transfer factor–current status and future prospects. Biotherapy 1996;9(1-3):1-5.

Leceta J, Gomariz RP, Martinez C, Carrion M, Arranz A, Juarranz Y. Vasocative intestinal peptide regulates Th17 function in autoimmune inflammation. Neuroimmunomodulation 2007;14:134-138.

Lenfant C. Clinical Research to Clinical Practice - Lost in Translation. New England Journal of Medicine 2003;349:868-874.

Leszek J, Inglot AD, Janusz M, Byczkiewicz F, Kiejna A, Georgiades J, Lisowski J. Colostrinin proline-rich polypeptide complex from ovine colostrum--a long-term study of its efficacy in Alzheimer's disease. Med Sci Monit. 2002;8(10):PI93-6.

Levine PH. The use of transfer factors in chronic fatigue syndrome: problems and prospects. Biotherapy 1996;9(1-3):77-79.

Lewis R. The rise of antibiotic-resistant infections. FDA Consumer – The Magazine of the U.S. Food and Drug Administration. 1995;29. (Accessed online July 25, 2007 at http://www.fda.gov/fdac/795_toc.html)

Li Q, Guo-Ross S, Lewis DV, Turner D, White AM, Wilson WA and Swartzwelder HS. Dietary prenatal choline supplementation enhances postnatal hippocampal structure and function. Journal of Neurophysiology 2004;41: 1545-1555.

Lim B et al Sunlight, tanning booths, and vitamin D. J Am Acad Dermatology. 2005;52(5); 868-876

Lombardi VC, Ruscetti FW, Das Gupta J, Pfost MA, Hagen KS, Peterson DL, Ruscetti SK, Bagni RK, Petrow-Sadowski C, Gold B, Dean M, Silverman RH, Mikovits JA. Detection of an Infectious Retrovirus, XMRV, in Blood Cells of Patients with Chronic Fatigue Syndrome. Science. 2009;326(5952):585-9.

Louie E, Borkowsky W, Klesius PH, Haynes TB, Gordon S, Bonk S, Lawrence HS. Treatment of cryptosporidiosis with oral bovine transfer factor. Clin Immunol Immunopathol. 1987;44(3):329-34.

MacDonald AB. Alzheimer's neuroborreliosis with trans-synaptic spread of infection and neurofibrillary tangles derived from intraneuronal spirochetes. Med Hypotheses. 2007;68(4):822-5.

Marshall TG, Marshall FE. Sarcoidosis succumbs to antibiotics – Implications for autoimmune disease. Autoimmun Rev 2004;3(4):295-300.

McCandless J. *Children with Starving Brains: A Medical Treatment Guide for Autism Spectrum Disorder*. New Jersey: Bramble, 2007.

McMeeking A, Borkowsky W, Klesius PH, Bonk S, Holzman RS, Lawrence HS. A controlled trial of bovine Dialyzable Leukocyte Extract for cryptosporidiosis in patients with AIDS. J Infect Dis. 1990;161(1):108-12.

Meduri R, Campos E, Scorolli L, De Vinci C, Pizza G, Viza D. Efficacy of transfer factor in treating patients with recurrent ocular herpes infections. Biotherapy. 1996;9:61-6.

Mead and Johnson. "Even closer to breast milk". (Accessed August 6, 2007 at http://www.enfamil.com/app/iwp/Content4.do?dm=enf&id=-8739)

Murillo-Rodriguez E, Haro R, Palomero-Rivero M, Millan-Aldaco D, Drucker-Colin R. Modafinil enhances extracellular levels of dopamine in the nucleus accumbens and increases wakefulness in rats. Behav Brain Res. 2007;176:353-7

NFID. Antimocrobial resistance. National Foundation for Infectious Diseases. 1997. (Accessed online July 25, 2007 at: http://www.nfid.org/factsheets/antimicrobial.html)

NIH. How HIV causes AIDS. National Institute of Allergy and Infectious Diseases, National Institutes of Health, US Department of Health and Human Services. November, 2004 (available online at:
http://www.niaid.nih.gov/factsheets/howhiv.htm).

Nishidaa A, Hisaokaa K, Zenshoa H, Uchitomib Y, Morinobuc S, Yamawakic S. Antidepressant drugs and cytokines in mood disorders. International Immunopharmacology. 2002;2(12):1619-1626.

Ojeda MO, Fernandez-Ortega C, Rosainz MJ. Dialyzable leukocyte extract suppresses the activity of essential transcription factors for HIV-1 gene expression in unstimulated MT-4 cells. Biochem Biophys Res Commun. 2000 Jul 14;273(3):1099-103.

Pardo CA, Vargas DL, Zimmerman AW. Immunity, neuroglia and neuroinflammation in autism. [International Review of Psychiatry. 2005;17(6):485-95.

Patarca-Monero R, Klimas NG, Fletcher MA. Immunotherapy of chronic fatigue syndrome: therapeutic interventions aimed at modulating the Th1/Th2 cytokine expression balance. Journal of Chronic Fatigue Syndrome. 2001;8: 3-37

Pilotti V, Mastrotilli M, Pizza G, De Vinci C, Busutti L, Palareti A, Gozzetti G, Cavallari A: Transfer factor as an adjuvant to non-small cell lung cancer (NSCLC) therapy. Biotherapy. 1996;9:117-121.

Pineda B, Estrada-Parra S, Pedraza-Medina B, Rodriguez-Ropon A, Perez R, Arrieta O. Interstitial transfer factor as adjuvant immunotherapy for experimental glioma. J Exp Clin Cancer Res. 2005;24(4):575-83.

Pizza G, Meduri R, De Vinci C, Scorolli L, Viza D. Transfer factor prevents relapses in herpes keratitis patients: a pilot study. Biotherapy. 1994;8(1):63-8.

Pizza G, Amadori M, Ablashi D, De Vinci C, Viza D. Cell mediated immunity to meet the avian influenza A (H5N1) challenge. Med Hypotheses. 2006;67(3):601-8.

Pizza G, Viza D, De Vinci C, Palareti A, Cuzzocrea D, Fornarola V, Baricordi R. Orally administered HSV-specific transfer factor (TF) prevents genital or labial herpes relapses. Biotherapy. 1996;9(1-3):67-72.

Popik P. Colostrinin and colostrinin-derived nonapeptide (colostral-val nonapeptide, CVNP) facilitate learning and memory in rats. Pol J Pharmacol. 2001;53(2):166-8.

Raqib R, Sarker P, Bergman P, Ara G, Lindh M, Sack, DA, Nasirul Islam KM, Gudmundsson GH, Andersson J, Agerbeth B. Improved outcome in shigellosis associated with butrate induction of an endogenous peptide antibiotic. Proc Natl Acad Sci USA. 2006;103(24):9178-83.

Raise E. Guerra L. Viza D. Pizza G. De Vinci C. Schiattone ML. Rocaccio L. Cicognani M. Preliminary results in HIV-1-infected patients treated with transfer factor (TF) and zidovudine (ZDV). Biotherapy. 1996;9(1-3):49-54.

Rocklin RE. Use of transfer factor in patients with depressed cellular immunity and chronic infection. Birth Defects: Original Article Series. 11(1):431-5, 1975.

Rubel J. Lyme Disease. Survival in Adverse Conditions. The strategy of morphological variation in Borrelia burgdorferi and other spirochetes. 1900-2001. September, 2003. (Accessed online January 11, 2009 at: http://www.lymeinfo.net/medical/LDAdverseConditions.pdf)

Russian Ministry of Health. Transfer Factors Use in Immunorehabilitation After Infectious-Inflammatory and Somatic Disease. Methodological Letter. Ministry of Health and Social Development of the Russian Federation, Moscow, 2004 (Accessed online January 11, 2009 at: http://russianhealthministry.blogspot.com/)

Rybakowski JK. Antiviral and immunomodulatory effect of lithium. Pharmacopsychiatry. 2000;33(5):159-64.

Samanek AJ et al   Estimates of beneficial and harmful sun exposure times during the year for major Australian population centres. Med J Australia. 2006;184:338-341.

Suarez EC, Krishnan RR, Lewis JG. The relation of severity of depressive symptoms to monocyte-associated proinflammatory cytokines and chemokines in apparently healthy men. Psychosomatic Med. 2003;65(3):362-8.

See D, Mason S, Roshan R. Increased tumor necrosis factor alpha (TNF-alpha) and natural killer cell (NK) function using an integrative approach in late stage cancers. Immunol Invest. 2002;31(2):137-53.

Siegel SD, Antoni MH, Fletcher MA, Maher K, Segota MC, Klimas N. Impaired natural immunity, cognitive dysfunction, and physical symptoms in patients with chronic fatigue syndrome: preliminary evidence for a subgroup? J Psychosom Res. 2006 Jun;60(6):559-66.

Schmidt-Wilcke et al   Striatal grey matter increase in patients suffering from fibromyalgia—A voxel-based morphometry study. Pain. 2007 Jun 21 (epub ahead of print)

Sokowlowska A, Bednarz R, Pacewicz M, Georgiades JA, Wilusz T, Polanowski A. Colostrum from different mammalian species – A rick source of colostrinin. International Dairy Journal. 2008;18(2):204-209.

Sperner-Unterweger B. Immunological aetiology of major psychiatric disorders: evidence and therapeutic implications. Drugs. 2005;65(11):1493-520.

Spitler LE. Transfer factor: failure to transfer reactivity in normal human subjects. Clin Exp Immunol. 1980;39(3):708-16.

Steele RW, Myers MG and Monroe VM. Transfer factor for the prevention of varicella-zoster infection in childhood leukemia. N Engl J Med 1980;303:355-359.

Steinman, L. A brief history of Th17, the first major revision in the Th1/Th2 hypothesis of T cell-mediated tissue damage. Nature Medicine 2007;13(2):139-145.

Stewart MG. Colostrinin: a naturally occurring compound derived from mammalian colostrum with efficacy in treatment of neurodegenerative diseases, including Alzheimer's. Expert Opin Pharmacother. 2008;9(14):2553-9.

Stewart MG, Banks D. Enhancement of long-term memory retention by Colostrinin in one-day-old chicks trained on a weak passive avoidance learning paradigm. Neurobiol Learn Mem. 2006;86(1):66-71.

Stiff, LA. Treating Chronically Ill Patients with Transfer Factor: An Exclusive Interview with Dr. Carol Ann Ryser, M.D. Originally published 10-31-2001. Accessed December 22, 2006 at http://www.prohealth.com/ /library/showArticle.cfm?libid=267

Szaniszlo P, German P, Hajas G, Saenz DN, Kruzel M, Boldogh I. New insights into clinical trial for Colostrinin in Alzheimer's disease. J Nutr Health Aging. 2009;13(3):235-41.

Time magazine, Monday, Dec. 30, 1974. "The Model Student". (Accessed January 10, 2009 at http://www.time.com/ time/magazine/article/0,9171,909028,00.html)

Tsao CW, Lin YS, Chen CC, Bai CH, Wu SR. Cytokines and serotonin transporter in patients with major depression. Prog Neuro-Psychopharm Biologic Psychiatry 2006;30:899-905.

Tupin E, Benhnia MR, Kinjo Y, Patsey R, Lena CJ, Haller MC, Caimano MJ, Imamura M, Wong CH, Crotty S, Radolf JD, Sellati TJ, Kronenberg M. NKT cells prevent chronic joint inflammation after infection with Borrelia burgdorferi. Proc Natl Acad Sci. 2008;105(50):19863-8.

Viza D, Vich JM, Phillips J et al Orally administered specific transfer factor for the treatment of herpesvirus infections. Lymphok Res 1985;4:27-30.

Wagner G, Knapp W, Gitsch E, Selander S. Transfer factor for adjuvant immunotherapy in cervical cancer. Cancer Detect Prev Suppl. 1987;1:373-6.

White AM. Why vaccines are not the answer - The failure of V520 and the importance of cell-mediated immunity in the fight against HIV/AIDS. Medical Hypotheses. 2008;71(6):909-913.

White AM. Could we reprogram the immune system to beat HIV without a bone marrow transplant from a donor with an anti-HIV gene configuration? Medical News Today. (Published online November 18, 2008 at www.medicalnewstoday.com/articles/129797.php)

White AM. Failure of the HIV-1 Step Study. Lancet. 2009;373:805.

Whitney D. Rapid spread of autism baffling. Sacremento Bee. November 21, 2003. (Accessed online July 25, 2007 at http://dwb.sacbee.com/content/news/story/7823487p-8764252c.html)

WHO. Nonpharmaceutical interventions for pandemic influenza, international measures. Emerging Infectious Diseases 2006; 12(1), 81-87.

Williams AC, Galley HF, Watt AM, Webster NR. Differential effects of three antibiotics on T helper cell cytokine expression. J Antimicrobial Chemotherapy. 2005;56:502-506.

Winkelmann RK, DeRemee RA, Ritts RE Jr. Treatment of varicella-zoster pneumonia with transfer factor. Cutis. 34(3):278-81, 1984.

Wolf JH. Low breastfeeding rates and public health in the United States. Am J Public Health. 2003;93(12): 2000–2010.

Wolf JH. Wolf responds. Am J Public Health 2004;94:1075-1076.

Wood et al Fibromyalgia patients who an abnormal dopamine response to pain. Eur J Neurosci. 2007;25:3576-82.

Yirmiya R. Depression in medical illness. West J Med. 2000; 173(5): 333–336.

Yirmiya R, Pollak Y, Morag M, Reichenberg A, Barak O, Avitsur R, Shavit Y, Ovadia H, Weidenfeld J, Morag A, Newman ME, Pollmacher T. Illness, cytokines, and depression. Ann N Y Acad Sci. 2000;917:478-87.

Xu YP, Zou WM, Zhan XJ, Yang SH, Xie DZ, Peng SL. Preparation and determination of immunological activities of anti-HBV egg yolk extraction. Cell Mol Immunol. 2006;3(1):67-71.

Zeisel SH. Nutritional importance of choline for brain development. J Am College Nutri. 2004;23:621S-626S.

Index

Appendix I

Abstracts of 160 studies spanning 60 years of research on transfer factors

In the years since Dr. Lawrence's discovery of transfer factor in 1949 and his initial publications on the topic in the mid 1950s, approximately 1000 articles were published in journals indexed by MedLine/PubMed (www.pubmed.gov). This was arrived at by searching MedLine/PubMed in December, 2008, for all manuscripts containing either "transfer factor" or "dialyzable leukocyte extract" and excluding those studies dealing with non-immune related research. For instance, the term "transfer factor" also has special meaning in lung research.

The list of abstracts was updated in December, 2009. At this time, the search was expanded to include "proline rich poylpeptides" and "colostrinin" as these appear to be synonymous with transfer factors. Only three papers using those search terms were included as examples (abstracts 158-160).

The present appendix includes the titles and abstracts of 160 manuscripts spanning 60 years. Papers are listed in chronological order of publication, allowing the reader to assess how the field of research on this topic has progressed.

The abstracts reflect both successes and failures. However, like the larger literature itself, more successes than failures are included. Manuscripts were chosen to represent the findings of research into various aspects of transfer factor activity, including their effectiveness in clinical trials involving various disease states in humans, work with in vitro preparations (i.e., studies involving the use of cells in culture), work involving laboratory animal models of disease states, and research into the molecular structure and mechanisms of action of transfer factors. Most review papers were excluded to focus on primary research.

Abstracts are numbered and an index is included to allow for quick access to findings relevant to the reader's topic of interest.

Index of select topics and abstract numbers

Numbered abstracts (in chronological order)

[1]

Lawrence HS. Pappenhiemer Jr AM. **Transfer of delayed hypersensitivity to diphtheria toxin in man.** The Journal of Experimental Medicine. 104:321-336, 1956.

Simultaneous transfer of delayed hypersensitivity to diphtheria toxin and to tuberculin has been accomplished in eight consecutive instances in man using extracts from washed leucocytes taken from the peripheral blood of tuberculin-positive, Schick-negative donors who were highly sensitive (i.e., pseudoreactors) to purified diphtheria toxin and toxoid. The leucocyte extracts used for transfer contained no detectable antitoxin. The recipient subjects were Schick-positive (<0.001 unit antitoxin per ml. serum) and tuberculin-negative at the time of transfer. All the recipients remained Schick-positive for at least 2 weeks following transfer and in every case their serum contained less than 0.001 units antitoxin at the time when they exhibited maximal skin reactivity to toxoid. Evidence is presented which indicates that the transfer factor may be released from leucocyte suspensions under mild conditions in which most of the cells appear to remain morphologically intact. Four adult Schick-positive subjects have been sensitized to diphtheria toxoid by intradermal injection of a few micrograms of purified toxoid in the form of a washed toxoid-antitoxin precipitate. Two of these sensitized individuals showed severe delayed skin reactions specifically directed against diphtheria toxin (or toxoid) at a time when their serum antitoxin level was less than 0.001 units/ml.

[2]

Shusuke T. Shunsaku O. Morio O. Takateru I. **Studies on the "Transfer Factor" of Tuberculin Hypersensitivity in Animals: I. Observation of Successful Passive Transfer of Tuberculin Hypersensitivity with Fractions of Either Disrupted Alveolar Macrophages or Serum of Sensitized and Challenged Rabbits.** J Immunol 93:838-849,1964.

Passive transfer of tuberculin hypersensitivity was accomplished with nonviable cellular constituents of alveolar macrophages of sensitized and challenged rabbits. Although cellular extracts *per se* had no activity to confer sensitivity on negative recipients, certain fractions obtained from them by electrophoresis, dialysis or treatment with ammonium sulfate, showed apparent activity to confer sensitivity. Thus, "transfer factor" is apparently present in rabbits as well as in man. "Transfer factor" is contained, but in inactive form, mainly in the supernatant fraction separated from particulate components of cells by 20,000 x G centrifugation. After dialysis of this supernatant, "transfer factor" appears in full activity. Dialyzed sera of sensitized and challenged rabbits also showed apparent activity to confer sensitivity, although serum *per se* had no activity. These facts led us to postulate the existence of a low molecular weight inhibitor. Reasons for these successes in effecting passive transfer with nonviable materials, despite many unsuccessful previous investigations in guinea pigs, have been discussed; in particular, the procedure of "challenge" by injecting BCG 4 days before harvesting the cells is thought to be very important for these positive results.

[3]

Kirkpatrick CH. Rich RR. Smith TK. **Effect of transfer factor on lympho-cyte function in anergic patients.** Journal of Clinical Investigation. 51(11):2948-58, 1972.

Dialyzable transfer factor, obtained from frozen-thawed peripheral blood leukocytes from a single donor, was given to five anergic patients with chronic mucocutaneous candidiasis. Studies of immunological responses including delayed cutaneous hypersensitivity, in vitro antigen-induced thymidine incorporation, and production of macrophage migration inhibition factor (MIF) were conducted both before and after injection of transfer factor.Before transfer factor, none of the patients had delayed skin responses to any of the natural antigens studied. Their lymphocytes did not produce MIF after exposure to antigens in vitro and only one patient showed increased thymidine incorporation when his lymphocytes were cultured with candida and streptokinase-streptodornase (SK-SD). After injection of transfer factor, four patients developed delayed skin responses to antigens to which the donor was sensitive; no recipient reacted to an antigen to which the donor was nonreactive. Lymphocytes from recipients produced MIF when cultured with antigens that evoked positive delayed skin tests. Only one patient developed antigen-induced lymphocyte transformation and this response occurred only intermittently. Attempts to sensitize three of the patients with the contact allergen, chlorodinitrobenzene, both before and after transfer factor, were unsuccessful.The fifth patient, a 9-yr old boy with an immunolog-ic profile similar to the Nezelof syndrome, did not become skin test-reactive or develop positive responses to the in vitro tests.These findings suggest that transfer factor acts on the immunocompetent cells that respond to antigens with lymphokine production, but has little, if any, effect on cells that respond to antigens by blastogenesis. The failure to sensitize the subjects with chlorodinitrobenzene illustrates the specificity of the immunologic effects of transfer factor, and implies that it does not function through nonspecific, adjuvant-like mechanisms. Failure of transfer factor to produce positive skin tests or MIF production in a patient with Nezelof's syndrome may be evidence that lymphokine-producing cells are thymus derived.

[4]

Spitler LE. Levin AS. Stites DP. Fudenberg HH. Pirofsky B. August CS. Stiehm ER. Hitzig WH. Gatti RA. **The Wiskott-Aldrich syndrome. Results of transfer factor therapy.** Journal of Clinical Investigation. 51(12):3216-24, 1972.

12 patients with Wiskott-Aldrich syndrome were treated with therapeutic doses of transfer factor in an attempt to induce cellular immunity. Clinical improvement was noted after transfer factor therapy in 7 of the 12 patients treated. Because this disease has a variable course and temporary spontaneous improvement can occur, the observed improvement cannot necessarily be attributed to the transfer factor. However, in two patients repeated remissions consistently followed transfer factor administration on repeated occasions. This included freedom from infections, regression of splenomegaly, and clearing of eczema. An unexpected finding was a decrease in bleeding in 3 of the 10 patients who had bleeding. Conversion of skin reactivity was obtained in all seven patients who clinically seemed to respond to transfer factor. In vitro studies performed after the administration of transfer factor demonstrated that the lymphocytes of the patients now produced migration inhibitory factor in response to appropriate test antigens, but did not undergo increased radioactive thymidine incorporation in response to the same antigens. A defect in the monocyte IgG receptors has been found in certain patients with the disease, and the current study shows that all patients with defective monocyte IgG receptors responded to transfer factor, whereas only one patient with normal receptors showed any response. This test may thus prove to be useful in predicting the results of transfer factor therapy in patients with Wiskott-Aldrich syndrome, although evaluation of a larger series of patients will be necessary to confirm this point. We conclude that cellular immunity can be induced, that there appears to be clinical benefit in certain patients with Wiskott-Aldrich syndrome by the use of transfer factor, and that this mode of therapy warrants trial in these patients and others with defects of cellular immunity.

[5]

Dressler D. Rosenfeld S. **On the chemical nature of transfer factor.** Proceedings of the National Academy of Sciences of the United States of America. 71(11):4429-34, 1974 Nov.

Two transfer factors prepared in an experimental animal model, the guinea pig, have been tested for their susceptibility to various enzymes of known specificity. The biological activity of these immune response mediators can be destroyed by RNase III, an enzyme that degrades duplex RNA. It, therefore, appears that these transfer factors consist entirely or partly of double-stranded RNA.

[6]

Oettgen HF. Old LJ. Farrow JH. Valentine FT. Lawrence HS. Thomas L. **Effects of dialyzable transfer factor in patients with breast cancer.** Proceedings of the National Academy of Sciences of the United States of America. 71(6):2319-23, 1974.

Five patients with advanced breast cancer were treated with pooled dialyzable transfer factor from healthy adult donors. The period of treatment ranged from 21 to 310 days, the total dose from 20 to 257 ml. Transfer factor did not elicit inflammatory or hypersensitivity reactions or detectable formation of antibody to itself, nor any hematological or biochemical abnormalities or other side effects. Three patients became responsive (by skin test) to tuberculin and/or streptococcal antigens. Marked partial regression of the breast cancer, lasting 6 months, was observed in one patient.

[7]

Zuckerman KS. Neidhart JA. Balcerzak SP. LoBuglio AF. **Immunologic specificity of transfer factor.** Journal of Clinical Investigation. 54(4):997-1000, 1974.

This study examined the immunologic specificity of transfer factor using a chromatographically purified transfer factor preparation. The specificity of transfer was examined utilizing immunity to keyhole limpet hemocyanin (KLH) and tuberculin. Transfer factor prepared from a donor immune to KLH successfully transferred KLH skin test reactivity to 10 out of 10 recipients. In contrast, comparable amounts of transfer factor from two donors not immune to KLH failed to transfer immunity to KLH in 11 recipients despite evidence for successful transfer of tuberculin reactivity. Unlike prior studies with a variety of antigens, the immunity to KLH in recipients of KLH immune transfer factor appeared comparable to that of the donor since both could be elicited with the same skin test antigen dose. These observations indicate that transfer factor can initiate a specific immune response to an antigen not previously encountered by the recipient and that in certain circumstances this immune response can be comparable to that of the donor. These observations on specificity and potency of transfer factor have important implications for the clinical use of this material.

[8]

Ascher MS. Schneider WJ. Valentine FT. Lawrence HS. **In vitro properties of leukocyte dialysates containing transfer factor.** Proceedings of the

National Academy of Sciences of the United States of America. 71(4):1178-82, 1974.

The chief impediment to the precise biochemical identification of transfer factor and its mechanism of action has been the lack of a reproducible in vitro assay. We now report on a method by which dialysates containing transfer factor of proven in vivo potency can convert nonimmune lymphocytes to immune responsiveness in vitro, as reflected by antigen-triggered lymphocyte proliferation. However, "water-dialyzed transfer factor" (TF(D)) prepared for in vivo use by the conventional method of dialysis against large volumes of water exhibits diminished activity in vitro and is frequently toxic to lymphocyte cultures. This problem can be avoided by dialysis of transfer factor into tissue culture medium. When this precaution is taken, such "media-dialyzed transfer factor" (TF(DM)) causes nonimmune lymphocytes to respond to antigen by an increment of thymidine incorporation that ranges from 2 to 25 times that of such cells cultured with antigen alone. This response is generally observed only in the presence of those antigens to which the TF(DM) donor expresses delayed cutaneous reactivity and is distinguishable from nonspecific adjuvant effects.

[9]

Jose DG. **Treatment of chronic muco-cutaneous candidiasis by lymphocyte transfer factor.** Australian & New Zealand Journal of Medicine. 5(4):318-23, 1975.

A beneficial clinical effect from the administration of lymphocyte transfer factor is described in six patients with idiopathic early onset chronic muco-cutaneous candidiasis. Five patients in two families showed a familial disease pattern. Dermal anergy and failure to produce migratory inhibition factor with intact general immune function were found in patients tested. Antifungal chemotherapy was effective in clearing or markedly reducing the candidiasis and remission was maintained by repeated injections of transfer factor. Therapy was monitored using Candida skin test.

[10]

Ng RP. Moran CJ. Alexopoulos CG. Bellingham AJ. **Transfer factor in Hodgkin's disease.** Lancet. 2(7941):901-3, 1975.

In a controlled studiy, six patients with stage-IV Hodgkin's disease were given transfer factor (T.F.) prepared from patients with Hodgkin's disease in long remission. There was an apparent increase in cell-mediated immune responses as evidenced by a significant increase in the recipients' lymphocyte responses to phytohaemagglutinin stimulation. Three out of six patients converted to positive delayed-hypersensitivity tests. These three all had the nodular sclerosing type of Hodgkin's disease. These results warrant the further investigation of the use of Hodgkin's disease-specific T.F. as a therapeutic agent in this condition.

[11]

Stevens DA. Ferrington RA. Merigan TC. Marinkovich VA. **Randomized trial of transfer factor treatment of human warts.** Clinical & Experimental Immunology. 21(3):520-4, 1975.

Dialysed transfer factor, prepared from the leucocytes of a donor whose warts had undergone recent spontaneous regression, was used in the treatment of a child with the Wiskott–Aldrich syndrome. The child then had a spontaneous regression at multiple warty areas. A similar relationship was seen in four otherwise healthy patients in a pilot study. A randomized double-blind study of thirty patients failed to confirm a causal relationship between the transfer factor therapy (equivalent to 2-1 X 10(8) leucocytes) and wart regressions. The need for randomized trials of transfer factor therapy for diseases with a variable natural history is emphasized.

[12]

Grob PJ. **Therapeutic use of transfer factor.** European Journal of Clinical Investigation. 5(1):33-43, 1975.

Transfer Factor (TF) was produced by ultrafiltration of repeatedly frozen and thawed, pooled buffy coats of healthy blood donors. One unit of TF Zurich was defined as the cell extract originating from 1 - 2 x 10-9 leucocytes. In collaboration with physicians and immunologists, 409 units TF have been given to 45 patients. Besides local pain and occasional fever no side effects were observed. Immune conversions and beneficial clinical effects were seen in 11 and 10 patients, respectively, out of 12 patients with chronic candidiasis. Immune conversion was also observed in patients with multiple sclerosis, while the clinical effects cannot yet be judged. The series also included patients with subacute sclerosing panencephalitis, HBAg-positive disorders, various immunodeficiency diseases, malignant malanoma and miscellaneous tumours. Immune conversion occurred only occasionally and the clinical effect was either non-existent or not judgeable. In the discussion the results of other investigators using TF therapy are included.

[13]

Kirkpatrick CH. **Properties and activities of transfer factor.** Journal of Allergy & Clinical Immunology. 55(6):411-21, 1975.

Although there is agreement that transfer factor endows skin test-negative subjects with the ability to develop the delayed allergic responses of the transfer factor donors, there is little direct information on the mechanism of this phenomenon or on the nature of the active components (s). This report reviews some of the known effects of transfer factor or immune responses and inflammation. It is concluded that transfer factor has multiple sites of action, including effects on the thymus, on lymphocyte-monocyte and/or lymphocyte-lymphocyte interactions, as well as direct effects on cells in inflammatory sites. It is also suggested that the "specificity" of transfer factor is determined by the immunologic status of the recipient rather than by informational molecules in the dialysates. Finally, it is proposed that many effects of transfer factor may be due to changes in intracellular cyclic nucleotide content, especially accumulation of cGMP, in immunologically reactive cells.

[14]

Rocklin RE. **Use of transfer factor in patients with depressed cellular immunity and chronic infection.** Birth Defects: Original Article Series. 11(1):431-5, 1975.

Two patients with chronic mucocutaneous candidiasis and a defect in cellular immunity received a single injection of dialysable transfer factor from Candida-positive donors in an effort to reconstitute immunologic function. The transfer of cellular hypersensitivity was successful in one of the two patients and was monitored by skin tests and MIF production; however, the effect was temporary and did not change the clinical course of the patient's infection. The other patient did not respond either immunologically or clinically to transfer factor at this time, although she did respond subsequently to repeated doses of transfer factor and amphotericin B therapy (Pabst and Swanson: Brit. med. J. 2:442, 1972). In another instance transfer factor from tuberculin-positive donors was used successfully to eradicate an infection in a patient with progressive primary tuberculosis and an acquired defect in cellular immunity. The patient had not responded clinically or bacteriologically after 7 1/2 months of antituberculous therapy, although the organism was shown to be sensitive in vitro to the drugs she was receiving. She received 6 doses of dialysable transfer factor over a 3-month period and during this time she responded clinically, bacteriologically and roentgeno-graphically.

[15]

Spitler LE. Levin AS. Fudenberg HH. **Transfer factor II: results of therapy.** Birth Defects: Original Article Series. 11(1):449-56, 1975.

Transfer factor is a dialyzable extract of sensitized leukocytes, which transfers reactivity from skin test-positive donors to skin test-negative recipients. Transfer factor supplied by our laboratory has been used therapeutically to induce cellular immunity in 78 patients around the world. Many patients received multiple doses of transfer factor ranging from 1 unit given every 6 months for 3 years to 1 unit every week for 6 months to as much as 8 units per week for a brief period. A total of 299 units of transfer factor have been given. Diseases in which transfer factor appeared to cause improvement include the Wiskott-Aldrich syndrome, severe combined immunodeficiency disease, mucocutaneous candidiasis, chronic active hepatitis, coccidioidmycosis, dysgammaglobulinemia, Behcet disease, aphthous stomatitis, linear morphea, familial keratoacanthoma and malignancy.

[16]
Vetto RM. Burger DR. Nolte JE. Vandenbark AA. Baker HW. **Transfer factor therapy in patients with cancer**. Cancer. 37(1):90-7, 1976.

The objective of this study was to utilize transfer factor to stimulate cell-mediated immunity to specific tumor antigens in cancer patients. Thirty-five selected patients with advanced recurrent cancer, who were not suitable for further conventional therapy, were treated with transfer factor. Transfer factor was prepared from cohabitants of the patients and administered at 2-week intervals. This immunotherapeutic approach produced a clinical effect in 13 patients in terms of regression of tumor (1), arrest of metastatic disease (14), or pain relief (14). Conversion of dermal reactivity to specific tumor antigens was observed during periods of clinical improvement. Despite continued immunotherapy, the duration of clinical improvement was short (2 weeks to 12 months). Seven of the 11 patients not responding to therapy exhibited serum blocking of lymphocyte responsiveness. In 11 patients there is insufficient data to evaluate the clinical effectiveness of this therapy. The results suggest that transfer factor can stimulate specific cell-mediated immunity in cancer patients and produce a clinical effect on tumor under certain circumstances.

[17]
Fudenberg HH. **Dialyzable transfer factor in the treatment of human osteosarcoma: an analytic review**. Annals of the New York Academy of Sciences. 277(00):545-57, 1976.

In conclusion, then, we would answer the seven questions raised earlier concerning transfer factor as follows: Certianly, as shown by clinical results, it does exist. It does have a definite immunologic effect in humans, boosting cell-mediated immunity, as shown by a rise in the level of active T cells. Its clinical effects have been demonstrated repeatedly, and it should become useful in still other clinical situations as further research provides more effective therapeutic modalities. Transfer factor from selected donors appears to provide prophylaxis against metastasis when administered to osteosarcoma patients with no clinically evident metastases at the time of surgical removal of the primary tumor; whether this treatment is superior to chemotherapeutic prophylaxis is conjectural and controversial. Its mechanism of action has not been demonstrated as yet, although many theories exist. The best evidence is that the effects are both specific and nonspecific. It appears to be produced by T lymphocytes. The exact nature of the substance we call "transfer factor" remains to be elucidated. Further research should provide more conclusive answers to these questions. [References: 51]

[18]

Ivins JC. Ritts RE. Pritchard DJ. Gilchrist GS. Miller GC. Taylor WF. **Transfer factor versus combination chemotherapy: a preliminary report of a randomized postsurgical adjuvant treatment study in osteogenic sarcoma.** Annals of the New York Academy of Sciences. 277(00):558-74, 1976.

Twenty-six patients with classic osteosarcoma were randomized to receive either transfer factor or combination chemotherapy. Eight of 14 patients who received transfer factor converted their skin test markers, evidence of activity of the transfer factor. Of these eight patients, all are alive; four are free of disease. Of the 18 patients who received combination chemotherapy, 14 are alive, 12 of whom are free of disease. The immunologic test procedures performed sequentially reveal that transfer factor appears to enhance cell-mediated immunity, but it is evident that in this study, a control (saline) arm in the protocol could not be included. It is of interest that the chemotherapy regimen used does not appear to suppress such activity permanently. The individual test results, however, are not very helpful for predicting response to treatment. The small numbers of patients and the short duration of this study, combined with the exclusion of parosteal osteogenic sarcomas and jaw tumors, do not permit a meaningful comparison with other published studies.

[19]

Goldenberg GJ. Brandes LJ. **In vivo and in vitro studies of immunotherapy of nasopharyngeal carcinoma with transfer factor.** Cancer Research. 36(2 pt 2):720-3, 1976.

Epstein-Barr virus, the apparent cause of infectious mononucleosis, may also be an etiological agent in nasopharyngeal carcinoma and Burkitt's lymphoma. Lymphocytes from normal individuals with anti-Epstein-Barr virus antibody activity may be sensitized to Epstein-Barr virus and contain transfer factor with the potential to program and/or recruit other lymphocytes to react against the virus and/or viral antigens. A patient with nasopharyngeal carcinoma refractory to conventional therapy was treated with transfer factor obtained from normal, young adults with previous history of infectious mononucleosis. Following immunotherapy, apparent slowing of tumor growth was observed, which was associated with intense lymphocytic infiltration of the tumor and reconstitution of delayed cutaneous hypersensitivity reactions to microbial recall antigens. A double-blind randomized clinical trial has been initiated to determine whether transfer factor immunotherapy is a useful adjunct to radiotherapy in the primary treatment of patients with nasopharyngeal carcinoma. If successful, a similar trial might be considered for African patients with Burkitt's lymphoma.

[20]
Behan PO. Durward WF. Melville ID. McGeorge AP. Behan WM. **Transfer-factor therapy in multiple sclerosis.** Lancet. 1(7967):988-90, 1976.

The effect of transfer factor prepared from relatives of patients with multiple sclerosis (M.S.) and from unrelated donors on the clinical course of M.S. has been studied in fifteen male and fifteen female patients. Some patients were given transfer factor and some placebo (physiological saline). Results of three independent clinical examinations by different neurologists and subjective assessments by the patients showed no difference between those given transfer factor and those given placebo.

[21]
Jersild C. Platz P. Thomsen M. Dupont B. Svejgaard A. Ciongoli AK. Fog T. Grob P. **Transfer factor treatment of patients with multuple sclerosis. I. Preliminary report of changes in immunological parameters.** Scandinavian Journal of Immunology. 5(1-2):141-8, 1976.

In five patients with definite multiple sclerosis and lack of cell-mediated immunity to measles and parainfluenza virus antigens, various immunological parameters were studied before and during transfer factor treatment. The study showed that cell-mediated immunity to measles virus antigen, as evaluated by the leukocyte migration agarose test, could temporarily be restored, using repeated injections of transfer factor pooled from unselected, normal blood donors.

[22]
LoBuglio AF. Neidhart JA. **Transfer factor: a potential agent for cancer therapy.** Medical Clinics of North America. 60(3):585-90, 1976.

This review has attempted to describe the characteristics of transfer factor which make it a very attractive potential agent for immunotherapy. Preliminary observations suggest that it may be capable of modifying resistance to a variety of diseases including cancer but considerable progress in basic knowledge regarding this agent is crucial to its successful application in clinical disease states. Fortunately, a sizable number of interested and dedicated investigators are exploring these difficult problems and their success may lead to new approaches in immunotherapy.

[23]

Horsmanheimo M. Krohn K. Virolainen M. **Clinical study of a patient with lupus vulgaris before and after injection of dialyzable transfer factor.** Journal of Investigative Dermatology. 68(1):10-5, 1977.

This report describes the clinical improvement and acquisition of tuberculin skin-test sensitivity by a tuberculin-negative, drug-resistant patient with lupus vulgaris after a single injection of dialyzable transfer factor (TFd) from a tuberculin-positive healthy donor. The patient's lymphocytes showed a slight response to tuberculin in the leukocyte migration inhibition test and in the lymphocyte transformation test before TFd injection. The acquisition of cellular immunity to tuberculin was demonstrated in vitro by enhanced tuberculin-induced blast transformation. A good correlation between skin test and in vitro tuberculin sensitivity and clinical improvement was seen during the three years that the patient was observed.

[24]

Grohn P. **Transfer factor in chronic and recurrent respiratory tract infections in children.** Acta Paediatrica Scandinavica. 66(2):211-7, 1977.

Five cases with abnormal sensitivity to respiratory tract infections are described. The cases showed a marked impairment in their cell mediated immunity state. Administration of a chromatographically purified transfer factor component increased the skin test sensitivity to common recall antigens. Interestingly, a similar effect in skin reactivity was observed with repeated skin tests alone, when antigen concentrations, initially high enough to cause a positive reaction, were used. Neither the administration of transfer factor nor skin testing with high antigen concentrations had an effect on blast transformation percentages. The therapy with chromatographically purified transfer factor appeared promising on the clinical condition of the patients.

[25]

Anttila R. Grohn P. Krohn K. **Transfer factor and cellular immune response in urinary tract infections in children.** Acta Paediatrica Scandinavica. 66(2):219-24, 1977.

Cellular immune responses in vivo and in vitro were studied in 20 children with chronic or relapsing urinary tract infections. Skin tests revealed decreased immune responses to PPD in cases with chronic or recurrent pyelonephritis and to OM, in these cases and in cases of lower urinary tract infections. Blast transformation responses to PPD, OM and PHA were at least as high as in controls. Administration of chromatographically purified fraction from human leucocyte transfer factor resulted in a positive skin reaction with antigen concentration, which before TF administration had caused a negative reaction. The results suggest that the action of the transfer factor component used in this study is based on an immunologically nonspecific stimulation of the cellular immune response.

[26]

Espanol T. Padulles J. Prats J. **Neuroblastoma and transfer factor.** Developments in Biological Standardization. 38:331-3, 1977.

Some authors have demonstrated the cytotoxic capacity of the mother's lymphocytes against the neuroblastoma cells of the son. It is not known if that is the reason for the better prognosis of these tumors in early infancy, and it was decided to treat some similar patients with transfer factor from the mother. The conditions for the patients were: more than 2 years old, poor response to chemotherapy and/or part of the tumor not resected. 3 to 5 doses of transfer factor were administered to 3 patients 2 1/2, 4 and 6 years old. One dose was taken from 400 ml of blood and prepared as described in the literature. The patients remained without metastasis more than 1 year after the treatment.

[27]

Kind CH. Gartmann JC. Grob PJ. **Transfer factor therapy in a patient with anergic pulmonary tuberculosis.** Schweizerische Medizinische Wochenschrift. Journal Suisse de Medecine. 107(48):1742-3, 1977.

Report on a patient suffering from severe, relapsing pulmonary tuberculosis showing progressive clinical deterioration accompanied by the appearance of cutaneous anergy to tuberculin. In addition, the sputum cultures showed growth of Mycobacterium intracellulare. During therapy with transferfactorZurich there was a slow but impressive clinical improvement, the skin reactivity to tuberculin was reconstitued and the sputum cultures became negative. The radiological findings remained unchanged.

[28]

Wolf RE. Fudenberg HH. Welch TM. Spitler LE. Ziff M. **Treatment of Bechcet's syndrome with transfer factor.** JAMA. 238(8):869-71, 1977.

Six patients with Behcet's syndrome were treated with transfer factor (TF) from randomly selected donors. Mucocutaneous symptoms and signs were predominant at the time that TF injections were started. Three patients showed great improvement, one moderate improvement, and one was unresponsive to multiple injections of TF from different donors. One case was uninterpretable because of concomitant administration of high doses of prednisone and chlorambucil and brief treatment with TF. These results indicate that TF therapy may be beneficial in some patients with Behcet's syndrome and that a trial of TF is warranted at least in the absence of severe ocular or neurologic manifestations.

[29]

Thulin H. Ellegaard J. Thestrup-Pedersen K. Zachariae H. **Long-term transfer factor treatment in severe atopic dermatitis.** Acta Allergologica. 32(4):236-7, 1977.

Transfer factor therapy was applied in three patients with severe atopic dermatitis and given at regular intervals for 1 1/2 years. Clinically, slight improvements were seen, attacks of impetigo ceased and admissions to hospital were not necessary. However, IgE concentrations in serum remained constantly high in all cases and the absolute number of T and B lymphocytes was continuously subnormal despite treatment. The in vitro cellular reactivity to PPD as assayed by a leucocyte migration test was not significantly altered in the patients, although a slight increase was found early on in the therapy. Finally, a serum factor inhibiting leucocyte migration and appearing simultaneously with attacks of impetigo disappeared during treatment. In conclusion, no convincing effect of transfer factor therapy was encountered in immune parameters and no major alterations were found in the status of the patients' atopic dermatitis.

[30]

Collins RC. Espinoza LR. Plank CR. Ebers GC. Rosenberg RA. Zabriskie JB. **A double-blind trial of transfer factor vs placebo in multiple sclerosis patients.** Clinical & Experimental Immunology. 33(1):1-11, 1978.

A double-blind trial of the effect of transfer factor on multiple sclerosis patients was carried out. In a series of fifty-six multiple sclerosis patients treated with monthly injections of either transfer factor or placebo for 1 year, no beneficial effect of transfer factor was noted. In addition, none of the immunological and serological parameters studied (measles migration inhibition, measles HI titre or CSF immunoglobulin) changed as a result of transfer factor therapy. Histocompatibility typing and CSF IgG/TP ratios were correlated with the disease activity. Of interest was the finding that the presence of the DW2 antigen, when unassociated with HLA-B7 antigen, appeared to correlate with the mildest form of disease activity.

[31]

Gross PA. Patel C. Spitler LE. **Disseminated Cryptococcus treated with transfer factor.** JAMA. 240(22):2460-2, 1978.

Cardiac toxic reactions and pulmonary consolidation in the left lower lobe developed in a patient who was receiving amphotericin B therapy for cryptococcal meningitis. Following surgical resection of the lobe, multiple subcutaneous cryptococcal abscesses appeared. Flucytosine administered intravenously failed to eradicate the lesions. Transfer factor therapy and multiple drainage procedures elimniated the skin abscesses. Transfer factor therapy was administered for one year; the patient was asymptomatic 16 months after therapy was discontinued.

[32]
Krown SE. Pinsky CM. Hirshaut Y. Hansen JA. Oettgen HF. **Effects of transfer factor in patients with advanced cancer.** Journal of Medical Sciences. 14(10):1026-38, 1978.

Eighteen patients with advanced cancer were given subcutaneous injections of pooled dialyzable transfer factor (TFd) from normal donors for periods of from 9 days to 6.5 months. Minor tumor regression was observed in only two patients, an effect of no therapeutic significance. However, treatment with TFd was associated with at least a temporary increase in delayed hypersensitivity reactions in 12 of 17 patients tested, including four patients who became responsive to 2,4-dinitrochlorobenzene. In general, in vitro tests of immune function were not changed after treatment with TFd except for levels of C1q, and/or C3, which were increased in 6 of 10 patients tested. We conclude that TFd may augment delayed hypersensitivity in patients with advanced cancer, and that its effects are, at least in part, immunologically nonsepcific.

[33]
Salaman MR. **An investigation into the antigen-specificity of transfer factor in its stimulatory action on lymphocyte transformation.** Immunology. 35(2):247-56, 1978.

Dialysable transfer factor (TF) was prepared from the buffy-coat cells of donors with known cell-mediated reactivity to tuberculin (PPD), streptococcal protein (SKSD) and diphtheria toxoid (DT). The effect of such preparations on the transformation by these antigens of lymphocytes from tuberculin-negative donors was investigated. Transformation was determined as incorporation of tritiated thymidine. The concentrations of SKSD and DT were adjusted for different lymphocyte donors so as to give, in the absence of TF, a low index of transformation (less than 10-fold) comparable to that obtained with PPD. TF from tuberculin-positive donors stimulated antigen-induced transformation by on average approximately 2-fold whereas TF from tuberculin-negative donors generally had little effect. This was so not for PPD as antigen but also for SKSD and DT, and sensitivity of TF donor to SKSD of DT was not a determining factor. TF also frequently increased background transformation in the absence of antigen. Although a small effect, this ability tended to reflect the activity of TF in the presence of antigen. It is concluded that neither the whole nor any significant part of this enhancement of transformation can be ascribed to an antigen-specific factor. Tuberculin-positive donors apparently yield a higher level of non-specific factor and possible reasons for this are discussed. The factor active in transformation may be responsbile for the TF phenomenon in vivo.

[34]

Grohn P. Kuokkanen K. Krohn K. **The effect of transfer factor on cystic acne.** Acta Dermato-Venereologica. 58(2):153-5, 1978.

A chromatographically purified component of human dialysable transfer factor, previously described as causing a non-specific stimulation of cell-mediated immunity, was used as a therapeutic agent in three cases of stage IV cystic acne. The treatment caused a marked strengthening of skin test responses and had a promising effect on skin eruption in each case.

[35]

Khan A. Sellars W. Grater W. Graham MF. Pflanzer J. Antonetti A. Bailey J. Hill NO. **The usefulness of transfer factor in asthma associated with frequent infections.** Annals of Allergy. 40(4):229-32, 1978.

Fifteen patients underwent controlled trial with transfer factor for repeated infections and severe asthma. Marked decrease in respiratory infections and striking improvement in asthma resulted. The authors suggest that transfer factor may reconstitute immune function, thus representing a unique approach to severe asthma associated with frequent infections.

[36]

Fog T. Pedersen L. Raun NE. Kam-Hansen S. Mellerup E. Platz P. Ryder LP. Jakobsen BK. Grob P. **Long-term transfer-factor treatment for multiple sclerosis.** Lancet. 1(8069):851-3, 1978.

In groups of 16 patients with multiple sclerosis, 13 months' double-blind treatment with transfer factor from random normal donors differed from placebo treatment only in producing a temporary restoration of lymphocyte reactivity to measles virus antigen, and did not arrest the degeneration of nerve tissue.

[37]

Hoyeraal HM. Froland SS. Salvesen CF. Munthe E. Natvig JB. Kass E. Blichfeldt P. Hegna TM. Revlem E. Sandstad B. Hjort NL. **No effect of transfer factor in juvenile rheumatoid arthritis by double-blind trial.** Annals of the Rheumatic Diseases. 37(2):175-9, 1978.

A previously pilot study of treatment with transfer factor in 3 patients with juvenile rheumatoid arthritis (JRA) gave promising results. However, in this small and open study no definite conclusions could be drawn. Therefore, a double-blind group trial was performed in 12 JRA patients treated with transfer factor, and in 12 placebo-treated control patients. The patients were evaluated clinically, by laboratory tests, and by estimation of different lymphocyte populations and cell-mediated immunity in vitro and in vivo. Transfer factor was not found to be of significant therapeutic value in patients with JRA. The only statistically significant difference between the two groups was a greater reduction in the percentage of T lymphocytes in transfer factor-treated patients than in control patients. The significance of this is difficult to explain and could have appeared by chance. No side effects of treatment with transfer factor were noted.

[38]

Ketchel SJ. Rodriguez V. Stone A. Gutterman JU. **A study of transfer factor for opportunistic infections in cancer patients.** Medical & Pediatric Oncology. 6(4):295-301, 1979.

Although supportive care during therapy of patients with malignancies has improved, infection remains the major cause of death in these patients. The problem of "opportunistic" infections is becoming more apparent as better antibiotics are found. The control of these infections depends in part on mechanisms of cell-mediated immunity. It has been demonstrated that delayed-type hypersensitivity can be transferred from one person to another. Therefore, we used transfer factor in the treatment of 15 patients, most with leukemia, who had fungal, viral, or mycobacterial infections that were not responding to conventional therapy. Seven of ten evaluable patients had therapeutic control of their infections while receiving transfer factor. Transfer factor appears to have contributed to these clinical improvements and is a modality of treatment that deserves further investigation.

[39]

Spitler LE. **Transfer factor in immunodeficiency diseases.** Annals of the New York Academy of Sciences. 332:228-35, 1979.

Results of therapeutic trials of transfer factor in a number of laboratories suggest clinical benefit and enhancement of immunological reactivity in patients with primary or secondary immunodeficiency diseases. Long term follow-up of 32 patients with the Wiskott-Aldrich syndrome suggested that transfer factor caused conversion of immunologic reactivity, apparent clinical benefit, and prolonged survival in some, but not in all patients. In 18 patients with disseminated (Stage III) malignant melanoma treated with surgery and transfer factor, survival was better than would ordinarily be expected for disseminated disease (78% with mean follow-up of 2 years). A randomized trial has been initiated which will answer the question of the efficacy of transfer factor as surgical adjuvant therapy in malignant melanoma. Studies in human subjects suggested that transfer factor does not cause enhancement of reactivity in normal subjects, when evaluated in a controlled, double-blind fashion. Similar controlled studies in immunodeficient patients are necessary to ascertain whether transfer factor does cause enhancement of immune responses in these patients. Based on these observations, a guinea pig model was developed in which transfer factor caused abrogation of tolerance to ABA-Tyrosine.

[40]

Ellis-Pegler R. Sutherland DC. Douglas R. Woodfield DG. Wilson JD. **Transfer factor and hepatitis B: a double blind study**. Clinical & Experimental Immunology. 36(2):221-6, 1979.

A prospective, double blind placebo-controlled trial was carried out on twenty-nine patients with hepatitis B. Thirteen received transfer factor and sixteen placebo. There were no significant differences between the two groups in any clinical or laboratory measurements made, although a rapid early reduction of serum aspartate transaminase levels by transfer factor is possible. Similarly, no significant changes were delineated by the in vitro measurements of lymphocyte function. Transfer factor did not alter the natural course of hepatitis B.

[41]

Faber WR. Leiker DL. Nengerman IM. Schellekens PT. **A placebo controlled clinical trial of transfer factor in lepromatous leprosy**. Clinical & Experimental Immunology. 35(1):45-52, 1979.

The effects of repeated injections of transfer factor over a period of 20 weeks were investigated in fourteen bacteriologically positive patients at the lepromatous side of the leprosy spectrum. All patients showed negative (0 mm induration) skin tests to M. leprae antigens (i.e. leprolin and lepromin). Of these patients, seven were treated with transfer factor with a total of 9 units (1 unit being equivalent to $5 \times 10(8)$ lymphocytes) and seven with a placebo. Maintenance treatment with clofazimine was continued. Transfer factor was prepared from the lymphocytes of donors who showed positive skin tests to M. leprae antigens (i.e. leprolin greater than or equal to 12 mm induration, average 15.5 mm or lepromin greater than or equal to 8 mm induration, average 13.6 mm), as well as a positive lymphocyte transformation in vitro to M. leprae (the average transformation being higher than the average transformation of lymphocytes of tuberculoid leprosy patients). No differences were found between the two groups as regards the clinical course of the disease, the histopathological and bacteriological evaluation of skin biopsies, changes in skin test reactivity to various antigens (i.e. lepromin, leprolin, PPD, Mumps, C. albicans, Tr. rubrum and Varidase), as well as the lymphocyte transformation in vitro to various mitogens (i.e. PHA, PWM, Con A) and antigens (i.e. M. leprae, leprolin, PPD, BCG, Mumps, C. albicans, Trichophyton and Varidase). No evidence was found to suggest that transfer factor is a valuable adjuvant in the treatment of lepromatous leprosy patients or that it increases cell-mediated immune reactivity towards M. leprae.

[42]

Spitler LE. Transfer factor therapy in the Wiskott-Aldrich syndrome. **Results of long-term follow-up in 32 patients.** American Journal of Medicine. 67(1):59-66, 1979.

Thirty-two patients with the Wiskott-Aldrich syndrome have been treated with transfer factor provided by this laboratory. Apparent clinical benefit was observed in 44 per cent of them. The mean age of the patients who showed clinical benefit was significantly greater than that of the patients who showed no benefit. Conversion of immunologic reactivity correlated with clinical benefit. Thirteen of the patients who received transfer factor are alive, and 17 have died (43 per cent survival). Clinical benefit was correlated with survival. The median survival was greater than five years in the patients who showed clinical benefit, whereas it was 18 months in those who did not show clinical benefit. We conclude that transfer factor caused conversion of immunologic parameters, apparent clinical benefit and prolonged survival in some, but not all, patients with the Wiskott-Aldrich syndrome.

[43]

Steele RW. Myers MG. Vincent MM. **Transfer factor for the prevention of varicella-zoster infection in childhood leukemia**. New England Journal of Medicine. 303(7):355-9, 1980.

Sixty-one patients with leukemia and no immunity to chickenpox were given dialyzable transfer factor or placebo and followed for 12 to 30 months in a double-blind trial designed to examine the clinical efficacy of transfer factor. Sixteen patients in the transfer-factor group and 15 in the placebo group were exposed to varicella zoster, and most of them had a rise in antibody titer. Chickenpox developed in 13 of 15 exposed patients in the placebo group but in only one of 16 in the transfer-factor group ($P = 1.3 \times 10^{(-5)}$). In the patients treated with transfer factor and exposed to varicella without acquiring chickenpox the titer of antibody to varicella zoster was equal to that in the patients given placebo who became infected with chickenpox. Transfer factor converted negative results on skin tests for varicella zoster to positive in approximately half the recipients. Passive immunization with dialyzable transfer factor appears useful in nonimmune persons.

[44]

Basten A. McLeod JG. Pollard JD. Walsh JC. Stewart GJ. Garrick R. Frith Van Der Brink CM. **Transfer factor in treatment of multiple sclerosis.** Lancet. 2(8201):931-4, 1980.

A 2-year prospective double-blind trial of the treatment of multiple sclerosis patients with the leucocyte extract, transfer factor (TF), obtained from leucocytes of relatives living with the patient, was conducted. 60 patients with definite MS, of whom 58 completed the trial, were divided into two equal groups, one of which received TF and the other placebo. The groups were evenly balanced with respect to sex ratios, disability, duration of disease, ratio of moderate to severe cases, and HLA phenotype. Neurological, electrophysiological, and immunological assessments were done at the start of the trial and every 6 months thereafter. The results indicated that (1) TF retarded but did not reverse progression of the disease; (2) a significant difference between treatment and placebo groups was not apparent with 18 months after the start of the trial; and (3) treatment was effective only in those patients with mild to moderate disease activity.

[45]

Khan A. Hansen B. Hill NO. Loeb E. Pardue AS. Hill JM. **Transfer factor in the treatment of herpes simplex types 1 and 2.** Dermatologica. 163(2):177-85, 1981.

Transfer factor potentiates cellular immunity and induces interferon. It was because of these properties that transfer factor was tried in 17 patients with recurrent herpes simplex types 1 and 2. Transfer factor was administered in doses ranging from 5 to 10 U/m2 i. m. The interval between injections varied from 1 week to 3 months. 16 patients could be evaluated clinically in whom the recurrence rate decreased from 10.7 +/- 6.1 to 2.1 +/- 2.5 (mean SD). The reduction was statistically significant. 8 patients were completely free of disease while the other 8 had reduced number of episodes during the period of observation, 7 patients had abnormal T cell function as reflected by the low number of T cells or low lymphocyte transformation. Statistically significant improvement in the T cell function was observed. Delayed hypersensitivity skin test reactions also improved significantly.

[46]

Lamoureux G. Cosgrove J. Duquette P. Lapierre Y. Jolicoeur R. Vanderland F. **A clinical and immunological study of the effects of transfer factor on multiple sclerosis patients.** Clinical & Experimental Immunology. 43(3):557-64, 1981.

A clinical and laboratory trial was designated to test the value of a potentially active pool of transfer factor (TF) given for a period of 3 months, at weekly intervals, in 27 relapsing MS patients and controls. The pool of TF was extracted from peripheral lymphocytes of 36 normal individuals presensitized with DNCB as marker. It was biologically capable of transferring DNCB sensitivity to MS recipients and did not show any toxicity. Clinically, a slight but not significant improvement of the functional and disability indices was observed in the TF group over a period of 1 year, while both indices increased in the control group. The treatment had no influence on the number of relapses and/or on sensory and visually evoked potentials, axial tomography and electronystagmography. In laboratory tests, a significant difference was found in the total CSF protein (P less than 0.05) and IgG (P less than 0.01) levels in the two groups studied; both values decreased or were stabilized in the group receiving TF, while they increased in the control group. Whether or not these slight clinically and biologically beneficial effects were due to the high dose of TF given or to its biological activity remains to be established. This pilot study suggests that a more appropriate answer regarding TF in MS might be obtained by using biologically active material, given for longer periods of time, at a closer interval and in a larger number of patients.

[47]

Jones JF. Minnich LL. Jeter WS. Pritchett RF. Fulginiti VA. Wedgwood RJ. **Treatment of childhood combined Epstein-Barr virus/cytomegalovirus infection with oral bovine transfer factor.** Lancet. 2(8238):122-4, 1981.

An illness lasting for two years, with recurrent fever, rash, abdominal pain, and arthralgia, developed in a four year old boy. He was found to have a combined Epstein-Barr virus and cytomegalovirus (CMV) infection. His symptoms, CMV in his urine, and an absent in vitro lymphocyte response to CMV antigen persisted for two years. After treatment with orally administered bovine transfer factor clinical symptoms and viruria disappeared and specific immunity to CMV developed. Evaluation of this treatment in chronic virus infections is warranted.

[48]

Blume MR. Rosenbaum EH. Cohen RJ. Gershow J. Glassberg AB. Shepley E. **Adjuvant immunotherapy of high risk stage I melanoma with transfer factor.** Cancer. 47(5):882-8, 1981.

Following conventional surgical management, 100 patients with high risk Stage I melanoma were treated with transfer factor to reduce the incidence of disease recurrence. All patients had primary lesions invasive to Clark's level III or deeper and exceeding 1.0 mm in measured thickness. Ninety-six patients are available for analysis at 15 to 67 months (median: 30 months) after diagnosis. Nine patients have had a recurrence of disease (treatment failure), and one has died. Actuarial non-failure rate is 90%, and survival rate is 99% at five years. A nonrandomized but contemporary control group of 46 patients displaying comparable risk factors was treated with surgery alone. The non-failure rate of this group is 63%, and the survival rate is 69%, data consistent with the results of several published studies. These results suggest that transfer factor immunotherapy may be a valuable adjunct in the treatment of patients with high risk Stage I melanoma.

[49]

Moulias, R. Lesourd, B. Hainaut, J. Marescot, M R. Epsztejn, M. Thiollet, M. Badoual, J. Reinert, P. Human **dialysable leucocyte extracts (transfer factor) in interstitial pneumonia. A retrospective trial in immunodeficient patients**. Journal of Clinical & Laboratory Immunology. 6(1):13-6, 1981.

Thirty-six cases of interstitial pneumonia in acquired immunodeficient states were treated with transfer factor (Dialysable Leukocyte Extract) and studied retrospectively. The criteria of efficacity of this treatment were: rapidity of immediate improvement, improvement after failure of other immunostimulant therapy and demonstration of a dose-related effect. The mechanism of the therapeutic action is unclear. There is no evidence in favour of "transfer" of cell mediated immunity. A non-specific mode of action (adjuvant effect, interferon synergy, proinflammatory action) seems much more likely.

[50]

Nekam K. Strelkauskas A J. Fudenberg H H. Donnan G G. Goust J M. **Evidence for the presence of a low molecular-weight activator of suppressor monocytes (LASM) in dialysates of T lymphocytes.** Immunology. 43(1):75-80, 1981.

Lysates of peripheral blood T lymphocytes from healthy individuals were found to contain a low molecular-weight peptide that inhibited phytohaemagglutinin-induced DNA synthesis in vitro by autologous or allogeneic peripheral blood mononuclear cells. The peptide was dialysable, partially heat stable, resistant to trypsin, RNase, and DNase but not to pronase, and was not part of the membrane receptor involved in rosette formation by T lymphocytes with sheep erythrocytes. It was found to act through monocytes, inducing the synthesis of second mediator responsible for the inhibition of lymphocyte DNA synthesis. This inducer of inhibition, designated as "low molecular-weight activator of suppressor monocytes' (LASM), may have a role in the depression of cellular immune response seen in various pathological conditions involving the destruction of T lymphocytes.

[51]

Jones, J F. Minnich, L L. Jeter, W S. Pritchett, R F. Fulginiti, V A. Wedgwood, R J. **Treatment of childhood combined Epstein-Barr virus/cytomegalovirus infection with oral bovine transfer factor.** Lancet. 2(8238):122-4, 1981.

An illness lasting for two years, with recurrent fever, rash, abdominal pain, and arthralgia, developed in a four year old boy. He was found to have a combined Epstein-Barr virus and cytomegalovirus (CMV) infection. His symptoms, CMV in his urine, and an absent in vitro lymphocyte response to CMV antigen persisted for two years. After treatment with orally administered bovine transfer factor clinical symptoms and viruria disappeared and specific immunity to CMV developed. Evaluation of this treatment in chronic virus infections is warranted.

[52]

Borkowsky W. Suleski P. Bhardwaj N. Lawrence H S. **Antigen-specific activity of murine leukocyte dialysates containing transfer factor on human leukocytes in the leukocyte migration inhibition (LMI) assay.** Journal of Immunology. 126(1):80-2, 1981.

We report on the extension of the direct leukocyte migration inhibition (LMI) test as an assay for antigen-specific activity in human leukocyte dialysates (DLE) containing transfer factor to an evaluation of antigen-specific activity in DLE prepared from inbred mice. Murine DLE was observed to cause antigen-dependent and antigen-specific effects on the inhibition of migration of nonimmune human leukocyte populations. Pulsing of nonimmune human leukocyte with DLE preparations from BALB/c and SJL mice immunized with Candida, diphtheria toxoid, and SK-SD resulted in their inhibition of migration in the presence of the respective antigens. The antigen-specific activity in murine DLE was found to be present in lymph node cell preparations and to be absent from spleen cell preparations of the same donors. The activity of DLE in lymph node cells was found to be present in the theta-cell enriched subpopulation of nonadherent lymphocytes after passage through nylon wool columns. The antigen-specific activity of murine DLE, as we have reported for human DLE, was found to reside in the < 3500 dalton dialysis fraction and not in the < 3500 dalton fraction. We conclude that nonimmune human leukocytes in the LMI test provide a suitable assay for the detection of antigen-specific activity in murine DLE as well as that in human DLE. Additionally, murine DLE is active across species barriers and appears to share properties with human DLE.

[53]

Thestrup-Pedersen K. Grunnet E. Zachariae H. **Transfer factor therapy in mycosis fungoides: a double-blind study.** Acta Dermato-Venereologica. 62(1):47-53, 1982.

Sixteen patients with mycosis fungoides (MF) were given either active transfer factor (TF) or heat-inactivated TF as additional therapy to topical nitrogen mustard or PUVA. The TF was prepared from non-selected healthy blood donors. The clinical evaluation after 2 years of therapy showed that among 8 patients treated with active TF, none went into complete remission of their disease 4 patients had partial remission, one was un-changed, 2 progressed, and one died of active MF. In the placebo-treated group, 5 patients achieved complete remission and 2 partial remission. One patient died early in the trial due to cardiac disease. Immunological studies during the first year of therapy revealed cutaneous anergy towards tuberculin in most patients. This anergy did not change during TF therapy and differed from normal lymphocyte reactivity in vitro after tuberculin stimulation. At the start of treatment the patients had diminished levels of T lymphocytes in peripheral blood. A temporary increase was observed in the total number of T lymphocytes in patients after one month of treatment with active TF. After one year the T lymphopenia had disappeared in both groups. The mitogen reactivity of lymphocytes was found to be normal (PHA, PWM) or somewhat reduced (Con A). It is concluded that under the conditions employed in this trial, TF was not able to prevent progression of early mycosis fungoides, when viewed over a period of 2 years.

[54]

Fujisawa T. Yamaguchi Y. **Transfer factor immunochemotherapy for primary lung cancer—evaluation of histologic types.** [Japanese] Gan No Rinsho - Japanese Journal of Cancer Clinics. 29(12):1409-16, 1983.

The clinical effect of leucocyte dialysate, including Transfer Factor (TF), on different histologic types of primary resected lung cancer was studied. This TF immunotherapy protocol included 171 patients. Eligible cases for evaluation were randomly chosen; the TF group and control group consisted of 75 and 74 patients, respectively. The TF group included 40 adenocarcinomas, 29 epidermoid carcinomas and 6 other histologic types of carcinoma. The control group included 42 adenocarcinomas, 25 epidermoid carcinomas and 7 other histologic types of carcinoma. The distribution of clinical features in the TF and control group was very similar, not only in adenocarcinoma but also in epidermoid carcinoma. The postoperative follow-up term was 2 to 55 months in both groups. Survival in the TF group of patients with adenocarcinoma of stages I + II or curative resection was significantly better than in the control group (p less than 0.005, Cox-Mantel test). There was no significant intergroup difference in patients with stages III + IV, relative curative or noncurative resection. Survival in the TF group of patients with epidermoid carcinoma of stages I + II or III + IV was about 20% better than in the control, however, there was no significant difference between the 2 groups. On the other hand, survival in the TF group of patients undergoing relative curative resection was significantly better than in the control (p less than 0.005, Cox-Mantel test). There was no significant difference among patients who underwent curative or noncurative resection. Time-versus-recurrence curves were evaluated by the Kaplan-Meier method; there was a significant difference between patients with stages I + II, but not between patients with stages III + IV. The frequency of recurrence of regional or intrapulmonary distant metastasis was lower in the TF group. It is suggested that TF suppresses postoperative recurrence and that it may be beneficial as postoperative adjuvant immunochemotherapy in primary resected lung cancer patients, especially those with relatively early stage cancer.

[55]

Fujisawa T. Yamaguchi Y. Kimura H. **Transfer factor in restoration of cell mediated immunity in lung cancer patients.** Japanese Journal of Surgery. 13(4):304-11, 1983.

We studied the transfer factor (TF) with regard to in vivo and in vitro restoration of cell mediated immunity (CMI) in lung cancer patients. Twenty-eight lung cancer patients who had undergone resection were the recipients and 30 household contact family members with a positive reactivity to lung cancer extract were the donors of TF. Immunologic status was evaluated by delayed type cutaneous hypersensitivity (DTH), peripheral T lymphocyte number, PHA lymphocyte blastogenesis, serum blocking activity (SBA) and leucocyte adherence inhibition (LAI) test. When TF was administered twice subcutaneously to the patients, there was a statistically significant restoration or augmentation of DTH, PHA lymphocyte blastogenesis and abrogation of SBA, particularly in patients with suppressed CMI. These results suggest that it was the TF obtained from relatives of lung cancer patients with positive reactivity to tumor associated antigens restored or augmented tumor specific and nonspecific CMI in these lung cancer patients.

[56]

Tanphaichitra D. **Cellular immunity in typhoid fever, Legionnaires' disease, amebiasis: role of transfer factor and Levamisole in typhoid fever.** Developments in Biological Standardization. 53:35-40, 1983.

Typhoid fever is an infectious disease commonly seen in the tropics, with multisystem involvement and a high morbidity and mortality rate. Legionnaires' disease: a newly described acute respiratory infection by unusual aerobic gram-negative micro-organisms namely Legionella pneumophila. Cellular immunity: in vitro and in vivo evaluations of cellular immunity using E-rosette formation (E) and 2.4-Dinitrochlorobenzene (D) reaction were made in typhoid fever, amebiasis and Legionnaires' disease. Results will be presented. Three patients with relapsing typhoid fever were given transfer factor and another group with typhoid fever were given Levamisole with sulfamethoxazole-trimethoprim. Up to 90% of the cases receiving immuno-potentiating factors/agents improved faster in both general condition, fever and cellular immunity.

[57]

Schindler TE. Venton DL. Baram P. **In vivo effects of human dialyzable leukocyte lysate. III. Modulation of the spleen cell proliferative response to antigen by components of leukocyte dialysates and an initial characterization of an ampliative nucleoside.** Cellular Immunology. 80(1):130-42, 1983.

The augmentative effects of isolated components of human dialyzable leukocyte lysates upon the proliferative response to antigen were investigated. Sequential Sephadex G-25 and Bio-Gel P-4 chromatography separated five distinct fractions which, 24 hr after injection into Keyhole limpet hemacyanin (KLH)-sensitive mice, either augmented or suppressed the in vitro spleen cell proliferative response to KLH. An amplifier molecule was isolated from one of the augmentative fractions by high-pressure, reverse-phase liquid chromatography. Preliminary structural analysis of the amplifier component indicated a nucleoside structure, similar to—but possibly distinct from—thymidine.

[58]

Dwyer JM. Gerstenhaber BJ. Dobuler KJ. **Clinical and immunologic response to antigen-specific transfer factor in drug-resistant infection with Mycobacterium xenopi.** American Journal of Medicine. 74(1):161-8, 1983.

The administration of transfer factor obtained from three donors who had recovered from clinical infections with Mycobacterium xenopi to a patient who had a destructive pulmonary infection with this organism, was associated with the reversal of an unfavorable clinical course. Cavitary tuberculosis associated with resistance to all combinations of antituberculosis drugs was probably related to a concurrent depression of cell-mediated immunity of unknown origin. Antigen specific but not nonspecific transfer factor caused a rapid and prolonged improvement in both the pulmonary disease and the immunologic deficiency. Cross-reactivity between the antigenic determinants of M. xenopi and Mycobacterium tuberculosis made it possible to use transfer factor obtained from donors responsive to purified protein derivative of tuberculin. This study clearly demonstrates the additional benefits to be gained from using transfer factor that is antigen-specific in the treatment of infectious diseases.

[59]

Fujisawa T. Yamaguchi Y. Kimura, H. **Transfer factor in restoration of cell mediated immunity in lung cancer patients.** Japanese Journal of Surgery. 13(4):304-11, 1983.

We studied the transfer factor (TF) with regard to in vivo and in vitro restoration of cell mediated immunity (CMI) in lung cancer patients. Twenty-eight lung cancer patients who had undergone resection were the recipients and 30 household contact family members with a positive reactivity to lung cancer extract were the donors of TF. Immunologic status was evaluated by delayed type cutaneous hypersensitivity (DTH), peripheral T lymphocyte number, PHA lymphocyte blastogenesis, serum blocking activity (SBA) and leucocyte adherence inhibition (LAI) test. When TF was administered twice subcutaneously to the patients, there was a statistically significant restoration or augmentation of DTH, PHA lymphocyte blastogenesis and abrogation of SBA, particularly in patients with suppressed CMI. These results suggest that it was the TF obtained from relatives of lung cancer patients with positive reactivity to tumor associated antigens restored or augmented tumor specific and nonspecific CMI in these lung cancer patients.

[60]

Dwyer J M. Gerstenhaber B J. Dobuler K J. **Clinical and immunologic response to antigen-specific transfer factor in drug-resistant infection with Mycobacterium xenopi.** American Journal of Medicine. 74(1):161-8, 1983.

The administration of transfer factor obtained from three donors who had recovered from clinical infections with Mycobacterium xenopi to a patient who had a destructive pulmonary infection with this organism, was associated with the reversal of an unfavorable clinical course. Cavitary tuberculosis associated with resistance to all combinations of antituberculosis drugs was probably related to a concurrent depression of cell-mediated immunity of unknown origin. Antigen specific but not nonspecific transfer factor caused a rapid and prolonged improvement in both the pulmonary disease and the immunologic deficiency. Cross-reactivity between the antigenic determinants of M. xenopi and Mycobacterium tuberculosis made it possible to use transfer factor obtained from donors responsive to purified protein derivative of tuberculin. This study clearly demonstrates the additional benefits to be gained from using transfer factor that is antigen-specific in the treatment of infectious diseases.

[61]
Kaminkova J. Lange CF. **Transfer factor and repeated otitis media.** Cellular Immunology. 89(1):259-64, 1984.

The effect of transfer factor (TF) was investigated in 12 children with repeated otitis media. These patients were immunologically compared to a control group of 23 age-matched healthy children. Levels of immunoglobulins, total and "active" T-cells, and phagocytic activity of granulocytes and monocytes were evaluated in the 12 children prior to, during, and after TF therapy. Percentages of "active" T cells and absolute numbers of "active" T and total T cells, which were initially low in the patient group, increased significantly after TF therapy to statistically match those of the healthy control group. The percentage of phagocytic monocytes in patients after therapy did not differ from healthy children; however, the percentage of phagocytic granulocytes remained depressed significantly. The levels of IgG, IgA, and IgM were unaffected by the therapy although the IgA and IgM were higher in the patient population throughout the study. After therapy, one-half of the patient population remained asymptomatic for a 1-year period and the others had markedly reduced attack rates.

[62]
Winkelmann RK. DeRemee RA. Ritts RE Jr. **Treatment of varicella-zoster pneumonia with transfer factor.** Cutis. 34(3):278-81, 1984.

A 29-year-old woman with a long history of immunoreactive disease—thrombocytopenic purpura, bullous pemphigoid, nephropathy, and hemolytic anemia—contracted generalized herpes zoster and varicella pneumonia. Respiratory failure requiring assisted respiration accompanied progressive chest findings. She recovered rapidly simultaneous with the administration of transfer factor from a healing herpes zoster patient. We believe that this therapy should be attempted in similar desperate circumstances.

[63]

Fujisawa T. Yamaguchi Y. Kimura H. Arita M. Shiba M. Baba M. **Randomized controlled trial of transfer factor immunochemotherapy as an adjunct to surgical treatment for primary adenocarcinoma of the lung.** Japanese Journal of Surgery. 14(6):452-8, 1984.

A total of 102 patients were studied in a randomized controlled trail to evaluate the clinical effect of transfer factor (TF) for primary resected adenocarcinoma of the lung. The TF and Control groups consisted of 50 and 52 randomly chosen patients, respectively. However, 6 and 5 patients were excluded from both groups for various reasons, therefore the total of cases eligible for evaluation were 44 and 47 in the TF and Control groups, respectively. The clinical features of both groups were similar. The survival of the TF group was significantly better than that of Controls in Stage I cases (p less than 0.05), however, there was no significant difference in patients in Stages II, III and IV. Significant differences were found between the TF and Control groups in curative resection cases (p less than 0.05), however, no significant difference was seen in either the relatively curative resection or noncurative resection groups. TF seems to inhibit postoperative recurrence and appears to be an effective postoperative adjuvant immunotherapeutic for primary resected adenocarcinoma of the lung, especially at the relatively early stages.

[64]

Kirsh MM. Orringer MB. McAuliffe S. Schork MA. Katz B. Silva J Jr. **Transfer factor in the treatment of carcinoma of the lung.** Annals of Thoracic Surgery. 38(2):140-5, 1984.

From 1976 to 1982, 63 patients with carcinoma of the lung underwent curative pulmonary resection, mediastinal lymph node dissection, and postoperative mediastinal irradiation when indicated. After operation, the patients were randomized by cell type and stage of disease into two groups. Beginning 1 month postoperatively, Group 1 patients (N = 28) received 1 ml of transfer factor that had been extracted from the blood of normal individuals. Subsequent doses were administered at 3-month intervals. Group 2 patients (N = 35) served as controls. There were no significant differences between the two groups with respect to age, sex, extent of resection, histological cell type, or stage of disease. Twenty of the 28 treated patients were alive and free from disease from 7 to 77 months after treatment, whereas 17 of the 35 control patients were free from disease. The 1-year survival for Group 1 was 84% and for Group 2, 81%. The 2-year survival was 78% for Group 1 and 46% for Group 2 (p = 0.045). The survival rates by stage of disease were as follows: Stage I, 15 out of 17 or 88% in Group 1 and 15 out of 23 or 65% in Group 2 (p = 0.097); Stages II and III, 5 out of 11 or 45% in Group 1 and

3 out of 12 or 25% in Group 2 (p = 0.304). The results of the study suggest that the administration of transfer factor to patients who have undergone pulmonary resection for carcinoma of the lung can have a significant impact on the prolongation of life.

[65]

Wilson GB. Fudenberg HH. Keller RH. **Guidelines for immunotherapy of antigen-specific defects with transfer factor.** Journal of Clinical & Laboratory Immunology. 13(2):51-8, 1984.

Dialyzable leukocyte extracts (DLE) containing transfer factor (TF) with documented specificity for one or more microbial antigens have shown previously variable clinical effectiveness in treating many infectious diseases caused by viruses, fungi, protozoa and mycobacteria. The efficacy has sometimes been strong, and at other times dubious, in treating patients with inherited or presumably "acquired" immunodeficiency diseases refractory to standard therapy. The recent development of assays for screening leukocyte donors of DLE, for monitoring recipients, and especially for determining the potency of various DLE preparations containing antigen-specific TF and for predicting the clinical course of disease have, in our hands, greatly improved the likelihood of successful immunotherapy with TF. Two representative cases are reported, one involving a patient with an antigen selective defect to Candida, and another involving a patient with an antigen selective defect to Mycobacterium fortuitum. Both patients responded as judged by laboratory tests and clinical improvement when treated with certain DLE preparations but not with others. Finally, certain DLE preparations appeared to suppress cell-mediated immunity in vivo and this suppression could be predicted by in vitro tests. Based on these results, guidelines for optimal therapy with DLE are proffered .

[66]

Zielinski CC. Savoini E. Ciotti M. Orani R. Konigswieser H. Eibl MM. **Dialyzable leukocyte extract (transfer factor) in the treatment of superinfected fistulating tuberculosis of the bone.** Cellular Immunology. 84(1):200-5, 1984.

The effect of the addition of dialyzable leukocyte extract (DLE)(transfer factor) to tuberculostatic drugs in the treatment of superinfected fistulating tuberculosis of bones and joints was evaluated in a controlled study. Eleven patients whose disease had persisted for a mean of 20 +/- 4.8 years and had proved to be resistant to antibiotics and tuberculostatic drugs were treated with an additional combined tuberculostatic drug regimen consisting of isoniazide, ethambutol, and rifampin for a control period of 2 years; after this therapy had failed as judged by the persistence of the superinfected fistulae and of the symptoms, DLE was added to the regimen. The result of this therapeutic approach was evaluated after another 2 years. Through this therapy, a closure of the fistulae was achieved in 9 out of the 11 patients (P less than 0.001) with a concomitant decrease of symptoms. DLE may prove beneficial in the treatment of patients with superinfected fistulating tuberculous osteomyelitis.

[67]

Borkowsky W. Martin D. Lawrence HS. **Juvenile laryngeal papillomatosis with pulmonary spread. Regression following transfer factor therapy.** American Journal of Diseases of Children. 138(7):667-9, 1984.

A 6-year-old girl with a history of juvenile laryngeal papillomatosis since 6 months of age and progressing pulmonary extension of the tumor for two years was treated with transfer factor prepared from her mother. Within one month of the onset of therapy, she exhibited marked clinical improvement. A computed tomographic scan performed after four months of therapy revealed almost complete resolution of her pulmonary lesions.

[68]

Fujisawa T. Yamaguchi Y. Kimura H. Arita M. Baba M. Shiba M. **Adjuvant immunotherapy of primary resected lung cancer with transfer factor.** Cancer. 54(4):663-9, 1984.

One hundred seventy-one patients were studied in order to evaluate the clinical efficacy of the transfer factor (TF) for primary resected lung cancers under a randomized controlled trial. Eligible cases for evaluation were randomly chosen at 75 and 74 patients in TF and control groups, respectively. The same long-term intermittent adjuvant chemotherapy was administered to two groups as a standard therapy. The distribution of clinical features in both groups was very similar. The overall survival rates of the TF group at 2 and 4 years postoperatively were 69% and 53%, respectively, which was about 15% better than the control group, but this difference could not yet be considered statistically significant. The survival of the TF group was significantly better than that of the control group in patients with Stages I + II or curative resection (P less than 0.05 by Cox-Mantel test); however, there was no significant difference in patients with Stages III + IV, or noncurative resection. The recurrence rate of pulmonary and mediastinal regions was less in the TF group. In conclusion, TF seems to suppress postoperative recurrence and appears to be beneficial for primary resected lung cancer patients, especially at early stages, as postoperative adjuvant immunotherapy.

[69]

Drews, J. **The experimental and clinical use of immune-modulating drugs in the prophylaxis and treatment of infections.** Infection. 13 Suppl 2:S241-50, 1985.

Therapeutic agents capable of stimulating immune responses could be of great value in the prophylaxis and treatment of infectious diseases. Three classes of compounds, each representing a separate approach to the goal of immune stimulation, are discussed with respect to recent experimental and clinical findings. The action of microbial structures and their derivatives can be understood on the basis of "acquired cellular immunity", a phenomenon first described in connection with infections by mycobacteria and other intracellular organisms. In contrast, there is hardly a common denominator for synthetic compounds which are currently used as immune-stimulatory agents. Substances which influence purine metabolism in lymphocytes on the one hand and histamine H2 blockers such as cimetidine on the other hand seem to represent the most promising developments in this field to date. Products of immune cells such as transfer factor and lymphokines form the third and possibly most important group of immune-stimulating agents. Current experimental and clinical trends in this field are briefly described. It is suggested that the delineation of the mechanism of action of lymphokines will open the door to the identification or synthesis of artificial agonists and antagonists as has been the case in the pharmacology of the endocrine and nervous systems.

[70]

Goldenberg GJ. Brandes LJ. Lau WH. Miller AB. Wall C. Ho JH. **Cooperative trial of immunotherapy for nasopharyngeal carcinoma with transfer factor from donors with Epstein-Barr virus antibody activity.** Cancer Treatment Reports. 69(7-8):761-7, 1985.

A prospectively randomized, double-blind clinical trial was conducted to evaluate the effect of immunotherapy with transfer factor (TF) as an adjunct to radiotherapy of patients with stage III nasopharyngeal carcinoma (NPC). The TF was derived from normal young adults with a proven history of infectious mononucleosis and from normal blood donors with elevated antiviral capsid antigen antibody activity. TF prepared in this fashion was previously shown to convert the leukocytes of patients with NPC to a reactive state in vitro and when administered to NPC patients in vivo was associated with apparent slowing of tumor growth, marked lymphocytic infiltration of the tumor, and reconstitution of delayed cutaneous hypersensitivity reactions. From 1974 to 1977, 100 patients with NPC were entered in the study; one-half of the patients were treated with radiotherapy alone and one-half received radiotherapy and an 18-month course of TF immunotherapy. The patients were followed for at least 5 years. No significant difference in disease-free survival or survival was noted between the two groups of patients. The use of this particular preparation and dose schedule of TF in patients with NPC with regional disease was devoid of any anti-tumor activity.

[71]

Georgescu C. **Effect of long-term therapy with transfer factor in rheuma-toid arthritis.**A Medecine Interne. 23(2):135-40, 1985.

Specific immunotherapy with transfer factor (TF) was used in a chronic experiment in a group of 50 female patients with rheumatoid arthritis (RA) stage I-III. The patients were followed up for 24 months, clinical and biologic examinations being repeated every 3 months. In this period the patients received beside the basic nonsteroid antiinflammatory therapy, one unit TF every week over a period of 6 months then one until TF every month (10 patients) to the end of experiment. Of the 50 patients 15 (30%) did not respond to the therapy and the experiments had to be interrupted after 6 months. Excellent, very good and good results were obtained in 35 patients (70%). In 12 patients the response was good but the dose of TF had to be increased to two units/week in the first 6 months. In 13 patients the results obtained were very good and therapy with nonsteroid products + TF was continued even after the first 6 months. In 10 patients with RA stage I the results obtained were excellent and after 6 months the nonsteroid therapy could be interrupted and the therapy was continued only with one unit TF every month. The study confirmed the fact that specific immunotherapy with TF represents an important adjuvant in the treatment of rheumatoid arthritis (RA).

[72]

Ashorn R. Uotila A. Kuokkanen K. Rasanen L. Karhumaki E. Krohn K. **Cellular immunity in acne vulgaris during transfer factor treatment.** Annals of Clinical Research. 17(4):152-5, 1985.

The effect of treatment with human dialyzable transfer factor was investigated on acne vulgaris patients in a double-blind study. About 1/3 of the patients improved clinically during the study period but there was no correlation between clinical improvement and transfer factor treatment. Prior to treatment parameters of cell-mediated immunity were significantly altered in the patients. These alterations normalized during the study in all patients irrespective of transfer factor treatment, possibly due to the immunostimula-tory effect of repeated skin testing. The present results support previous findings that acne patients have slightly altered cell-mediated immunity, but the results further suggest that abnormalities are not significant in the pathogenesis of acne vulgaris.

[73]

Li ZL. **The study of human transfer factor.** Scientia Sinica - Series B, Chemical, Biological, Agricultural, Medical & Earth Sciences. 28(4):394-401, 1985.

In this paper, the study of human transfer factor is reported. We established a negative pressure dialysis method instead of ordinary dialysis for treatment of the crude leukocyte extract. Dialysate is rapidly obtained in only 5 h so that a large volume of preparation is easier to handle and the chance of contamination avoided. When human TF was incubated with human cord blood T-lymphocytes and pig lymphocytes, a very high biological activity on SRBC rosette enhancement and an increase in electrophoresis rate appeared. It suggests that these assays may be used as in vitro method of evaluation of TF activity. In our clinic, TF has been in clinical trials for 5 years and has now been administered to a large number of patients with a variety of diseases, in which cell-mediated immune responses have been compromised. We observe that TF has served an efficient immunopotentiating or immunomodulation agent.

[74]

Roda E. Viza D. Pizza G. Mastroroberto L. Phillips J. De Vinci C. Barbara L. **Transfer factor for the treatment of HBsAg-positive chronic active hepatitis.** Proceedings of the Society for Experimental Biology & Medicine. 178(3):468-75, 1985.

Transfer factor was obtained from four patients having recovered from acute type-B viral hepatitis. It was replicated in vitro using the LDV/7 lymphoblastoid cell line. This in vitro-produced transfer factor specific for hepatitis B (TFdL-H) was administered to 10 randomly selected patients with biochemically and histologically proven HBsAg-positive chronic active hepatitis (CAH) at 15-day intervals over a 6-month period. In three out of four initially HBeAg-positive patients, anti-HBe antibodies appeared when the HBeAg disappeared. In one of these patients and in two other HBsAg-positive patients, the appearance of anti-HBs antibodies was noted. The improvement in several biochemical parameters of the TFdL-H patients was statistically significant when compared with those of another group of 10 randomly selected untreated CAH patients. Liver biopsies in six out of eight treated patients showed a histological improvement at the end of the treatment. These results suggest that TFdL-H may be used with beneficial effect for the treatment of HBsAg-positive CAH.

[75]

Tsang KY. Fudenberg HH. Pan JF. **Transfer of osteosarcoma-specific cell-mediated immunity in hamsters by rabbit dialyzable leukocyte extracts.** Cellular Immunology. 90(2):295-302, 1985.

We have investigated the transfer of specific cell-mediated immunity (CMI) to osteosarcoma-associated antigens (OSAA) to hamsters with dialyzable leukocyte extracts (DLE) from OSAA-immunized rabbits. The transfer of specific CMI was determined by leukocyte adherence inhibition (LAI) assay and skin testing. DLE was prepared from rabbits immunized with OSAA, purified protein derivative (PPD), or fibrosarcoma cell plasma membrane preparation (FSM). Control DLE was prepared from rabbits injected with 0.85% NaCl. Significant leukocyte adherence inhibition was observed with leukocytes from hamsters that had received OSAA-specific, PPD-specific, and FSM-specific rabbit DLE, when OSAA, PPD, and FSM were used as antigens, respectively. Similarly, significant ear swelling after injection of OSAA, PPD, or FSM was observed only in hamsters that had received DLE from rabbits immunized with OSAA, PPD, or FSM, respectively. These results suggest that CMI specific for OSAA, PPD, or FSM can be transferred to normal hamsters by DLE from immunized rabbits.

[76]

Frith JA. McLeod JG. Basten A. Pollard JD. Hammond SR. Williams DB. Crossie PA.**Transfer factor as a therapy for multiple sclerosis: a follow-up study.** Clinical & Experimental Neurology. 22:149-54, 1986.

The result of a two year, double blind, controlled trial of Transfer Factor (TF) in the treatment of multiple sclerosis (MS) were reported in 1980. It was demonstrated that TF significantly reduced the rate of progression of the disability but the benefit of therapy was not apparent until 18 months after its commencement. After the completion of the trial, TF treatment was offered to all the trial participants. Forty-five of these people accepted TF as treatment and have been followed for the subsequent three years. The twenty-three people who had received TF during the trial, and continued on TF after the trial, consistently had a slower rate of progression of their MS. Although the twenty-two patients initially on placebo had a significantly faster rate of progression during the trial, this slowed with commencement of TF treatment. After 3 years of TF, the rate of progression of disease was similar to that of the group receiving TF continuously for 5 years. In addition, 470 patients with clinically definite MS are being treated in New South Wales in an open study of TF. The rate of progression of the disease is being monitored by neurological assessments and appears to be similar to that of patients who had received TF in the original trial. The follow-up study of the 1980 TF trial patients and the open study of 470 MS patients confirm the original observation that TF has some effect on slowing the course of MS.

[77]

Van Haver H. Lissoir F. Droissart C. Ketelaer P. Van Hees J. Theys P. Vervliet G. Claeys H. Gautama K. Vermylen C. et al **Transfer factor therapy in multiple sclerosis: a three-year prospective double-blind clinical trial.** Neurology. 36(10):1399-402, 1986.

One hundred five patients with MS were divided into three groups matched for age, sex, and disability, and treated with either placebo, transfer factor prepared from leukocytes of random donors, or transfer factor from leukocytes of family members living with the patients. There were no differences in the three treatment groups for changes in disability, activities of daily living, or evoked potentials. Eighteen months of transfer factor therapy had no effect on gamma-interferon production or natural killer cell activities.

[78]

Viza D. Vich JM. Phillips J. Rosenfeld F. Davies DA. **Specific transfer factor protects mice against lethal challenge with herpes simplex virus.** Cellular Immunology. 100(2):555-62, 1986.

Bovine transfer factor (TFd) specific to herpes simplex virus (HSV)1 or to HSV2 was prepared by immunizing calves with the corresponding virus. The TFd preparations were then injected into Swiss mice in an attempt to protect them against a subsequent lethal challenge with HSV1 or HSV2 virus. It was thus shown that injection of anti-HSV TFd protects the mice against the corresponding HSV virus, whereas the injection of a nonspecific TFd (anti-CMV) fails to protect against a challenge with HSV1. Furthermore, a dose-response effect was observed, since potent TFd preparations were ineffective when they were used at one-fifth of the original concentration. It seems, therefore, that animal models may be used to assay the potency of TFd preparations specific for herpes viruses.

[79]

Spitler LE. Miller L. Paul M. **Clinical trials of transfer factor in malignancy.** Journal of Experimental Pathology. 3(4):549-64, 1987.

Results of clinical trials of transfer factor therapy in various malignancies have been variable. In non randomized trials, about 300 patients have been evaluated, and clinical benefit has been reported in about 1/3 of the evaluable patients. Results of randomized studies are similarly varied. In some randomized trials, clinical benefits of increased disease free survival and prolonged survival have been claimed. In other studies, transfer factor has been reported to be of no clinical benefit. In a few studies, results suggest patients receiving transfer factor do not do as well as those receiving placebo, although these are only trends, and do not reach the level of statistical significance. There are a number of variables in the design of transfer factor trials, and review of the studies performed to date does not permit a determination of which, if any, of these variables is related to the therapeutic outcome. A variety of tumor types have been evaluated, and it is not clear which, if any, tumors respond to transfer factor. Similarly, the state of disease and prior and concomitant therapy vary widely in these trials and the impact of these variables is unclear. The source and dose of transfer factor also varies. In some studies, attempts have been made to select donors who might have cellular immune reactivity to the tumor being treated, whereas in other studies normal donors have been used. The rationale for the use of normal donors in that the clinical benefit of transfer factor may be related to the non specific immunopotentiating effects of this agent rather than the specific transfer of cellular immunity. Finally, the methods of preparation of transfer factor vary and the products used in various studies cannot be compared by standard biologic or biochemical tests currently available. This review of the literature regarding the clinical effort of transfer factor in malignancy leads to the conclusion that transfer factor might not be an effective therapy of cancer. If it does have efficacy in certain malignancies, it is unlikely that it will alone have dramatic effects in substantial numbers of patients. Perhaps transfer factor may have a role in tumor therapy as an adjuvant to other forms of therapy and as surgery, irradiation, or chemotherapy. In order for the proper evaluation of transfer factor in reproducible comparative studies, it will be necessary to have a standarized reproducible product which can be assessed by appropriate quality control procedures.

[80]
Nkrumah FK. Pizza G. Neequaye J. Viza D. De Vinci C. Levine PH. **Transfer factor in prevention Burkitt's lymphoma relapses.** Journal of Experimental Pathology. 3(4):463-9, 1987.

Twenty-two African children with endemic Burkitt's lymphoma entered a study to evaluate the possible efficacy of a transfer factor (TF) with specific activity against Eptein-Barr virus in preventing disease relapses. Five of eleven patients have so far relapsed in the non TF-treated group as against two of eleven in the TF-treated group. The patterns of relapse and observable increased disease free remission duration in the TF-treated group strongly suggest a beneficial effect particularly in the prevention of late relapses. A larger series of patients treated with this specific TF are needed to confirm these observations in endemic Burkitt's lymphoma.

[81]

Huang LL. Su CZ. Wan ZF. **Nature and antigen-specific activities of transfer factor against herpes simplex virus type 1**. Acta Virologica. 31(6):449-57, 1987.

Transfer factor specific for herpes simplex virus (HSV) type 1 (TFHSV-1) was prepared from splenic cells of HSV-1 immunized mice. Protection was transferred with TFHSV-1 to nonimmune mouse recipients. The TFHSV-1 injected mice had a higher survival rate after lethal HSV-1 challenge as compared to mice injected with a nonspecific transfer factor (P less than 0.05). 51Cr-labelled leukocyte adherence inhibition (51-Cr-LAI) test was used to demonstrate the specific activity of transfer factor in vitro. Only leukocytes incubated with TFHSV-1 exhibited significant adherence inhibition (P less than 0.01) to HSV-1 antigen, but not to control antigen. Specific activity component of TFHSV-1 (STFc) was separated by affinity adsorption with the antigen. Activity of STFc in 51Cr-LAI test was significantly higher than that of TFHSV-1 (P less than 0.01). Ratio activity of STFc in protective host immunity was 16 times as much as that of TFHSV-1. STFc was analysed by high performance liquid chromatography, thin layer chromatography and isoelectric focusing in the polyacrylamide gel. Results revealed that STFc appeared to be a polypeptide with a molecular weight of about 12,870 dalton.

[82]

Wagner G. Knapp W. Gitsch E. Selander S. **Transfer factor for adjuvant immunotherapy in cervical cancer**. Cancer Detection & Prevention. Supplement. 1:373-6, 1987.

In a prospective randomized double-blind study of 60 patients with invasive cervical cancer, 32 were treated with transfer factor (TF) derived from leukocytes of the patients' husbands, and 28 were treated with placebo. Within the first 2 years after radical hysterectomy, five out of 32 TF-treated patients and 11 out of 28 placebo-treated patients developed recurrence of malignancy. Excluding one further patient with intercurrent death this difference is significant (chi 2 = 3.9915; P less than 0.05). Subdividing the collectives, significant differences were found in patients aged below 35 years and in patients with stage I disease. Identical immune profiles were checked in leukocyte donors prior to leukophoresis and were serially checked in patients. Antigen-specific correlations were found between donors' and recipients' reactivities but not between donors' reactivity and recipient's course of the disease.

[83]

Louie E. Borkowsky W. Klesius PH. Haynes TB. Gordon S. Bonk S. Lawrence HS. **Treatment of cryptosporidiosis with oral bovine transfer factor.** Clinical Immunology & Immunopathology. 44(3):329-34, 1987.

Cryptosporidia are intestinal protozoans long known to cause diarrhea in humans, especially those with acquired immune deficiency syndrome (AIDS). When transfer factor prepared from calves which possessed delayed-type hypersensitivity to Eimeria bovis was given to nonimmune calves and mice it conferred protection against clinical infection (coccidiosis). Recent studies with oral bovine transfer factor have shown that it can confer cell-mediated immunity to humans. Based on these findings we decided to treat eight AIDS patients suffering from Cryptosporidium-associated diarrhea with transfer factor prepared from calves immune to Cryptosporidium. Prior to treatment with transfer factor, three patients had been treated with spiramycin, one patient with alpha-difluoromethylornithine (DFMO), and one patient with furazolidone for greater than 1 month without clinical or laboratory improvement. Following administration of transfer factor, five or eight patients exhibited a decrease in the number of bowel movements and the development of formed stools. Cryptosporidium was eradicated from the stools of four patients but two of these patients subsequently relapsed and one patient continued to have diarrhea despite the absence of Cryptosporidium in the stool. One patient has been free of diarrhea and Cryptosporidium for 2 years after discontinuation of transfer factor therapy.

[84]

Carey, J T. Lederman, M M. Toossi, Z. Edmonds, K. Hodder, S. Calabrese, L H. Proffitt, M R. Johnson, C E. Ellner, J J. **Augmentation of skin test reactivity and lymphocyte blastogenesis in patients with AIDS treated with transfer factor.** JAMA. 257(5):651-5, 1987.

Nine patients with the acquired immunodeficiency syndrome (AIDS) were administered four doses of pooled transfer factor obtained from the lymphocytes of three healthy controls and three homosexuals with stable lymphadenopathy and serum antibody to the human immunodeficiency virus. Before receiving transfer factor, all patients exhibited anergy to skin test antigens. After four weeks of transfer factor therapy, six of seven patients tested had at least one skin test response. Lymphocyte blastogenic responses to phytohemagglutinin rose from a stimulation index of 6.77 +/- 1.31 before treatment to 19.77 +/- 6.24 after four weeks of transfer factor therapy. Smaller but significant increases were also seen in blastogenic responses to antigens. Improvements in immune responses diminished after administration of transfer factor was halted. Thus, administration of transfer factor to patients with AIDS resulted in partial immune reconstitution. Further studies are indicated to examine the clinical efficacy of this immune response modifier in the treatment of AIDS.

[85]

Waisbren BA Sr. **Observations on the combined systemic administration of mixed bacterial vaccine, bacillus Calmette-Guerin, transfer factor, and lymphoblastoid lymphocytes to patients with cancer, 1974-1985.** Journal of Biological Response Modifiers. 6(1):1-19, 1987.

Herein are reported the results of treating 139 cancer patients with combined immunomodulation that consisted of bacillus Calmette-Guerin, transfer factor, and mixed bacterial vaccine. In addition 28 patients were given infusions of lymphoblastoid lymphocytes. Patients were admitted to this treatment program who either had failed to respond to other modalities, had elected to add immunomodulation to usual therapy, or had refused chemotherapy and/or radiation therapy. The results suggested that combined immunomodulation therapy is well tolerated and safe and that this approach on a prima facie basis had a salutary effect on the courses of a number of the patients treated. The results also illustrate alternative pathways that can be taken by patients and physicians who are not comfortable with protocolized double-blind methods of approaching patients with poor prognosis cancer.

[85]

Tsang KY. Pan JF. Fudenberg HH. **An animal model for evaluation of antigen-specific dialyzable leukocyte extracts therapy of osteosarcoma.** Clinical Immunology & Immunopathology. 42(3):360-9, 1987.

The effects of human osteosarcoma (OS)-specific dialyzable leukocyte extracts (DLE) in hamsters bearing human OS were investigated. The DLE used in this investigation was prepared from rabbits immunized with human osteosarcoma-associated antigens (DLE-OSAA). Tuberculin (DLE-PPD) and control DLE were prepared from rabbits injected with tuberculin or 0.85% NaCl (DLE-NaCl). DLE was administered subcutaneously into inbred hamsters (each injection contained DLE derived from 10(7) rabbit leukocytes). Four groups of animals were studied: group 1, amputation alone; group 2, amputation plus DLE-OSAA; group 3, amputation plus DLE-PPD; group 4, amputation plus DLE-NaCl. Of the DLE-OSAA-treated animals (group 2), 60% were still alive at 300 days postamputation; whereas in animals in groups 1, 3, and 4, all died within 90 days postamputation. In separate experiments, we found that 100% of the animals in groups 1, 3, and 4 developed pulmonary metastases within 30-60 days postamputation, whereas only 20% of the animals in group 2 developed metastases at the same time; indeed 40% of the DLE-OSAA-treated animals were free of metastases in 240-300 days postamputation. Both the leukocyte adherence inhibition assay (LAI) and lymphocyte DNA synthesis assay (LDS) were used to monitor the transfer of antigen-specific cell-mediated immunity in each group of tumor-bearing hamsters. All surviving hamsters in group 2 had high LAI and LDS activity. Our results suggest that DLE-OSAA is effective in preventing pulmonary metastases and death of OS-bearing hamsters (after amputation) as compared with amputation alone, amputation plus DLE-NaCl, and amputation plus DLE-PPD, and that its effect is via an antigen-specific mechanism.

[87]

Hancock BW. Bruce L. Sokol RJ. Clark A. University Department of Medicine, Royal Hallamshire Hospital, Sheffield, U.K. **Transfer factor in Hodgkin's disease: a randomized clinical and immunological study.** European Journal of Cancer & Clinical Oncology. 24(5):929-33, 1988.

Transfer factor (TF) was prepared from buffy coats obtained from 493 units of blood taken from healthy donors, including individuals convalescent from various viral infections. It was administered to 22 of 47 patients with Hodgkin's disease undergoing treatment and consenting to take part in this randomized study to determine if TF would enhance their immunity and/or reduce the incidence of subsequent infections. Skin test reactivity was markedly enhanced in those patients receiving TF as opposed to placebo but other immunological assessments showed no significant differences between the groups. TF was not shown to be of benefit in the prevention of infections (including varicella/zoster).

[88]

Lukacs, K. Szabo, G. Schroder, I. Szegedi, G. **Adult chronic granulomatosis disease-like neutrophil granulocyte disorder corrected by dialysable leukocyte extract.** Allergologia et Immunopathologia. 16(2):121-5, 1988.

A 47 year old female presented with a septic clinical picture including fever, abscesses, late cachexia, and unmanageable by disease. Similar characteristics to chronic granulomatosis disease (CGD) seriously decreased intracellular killing activity and chemiluminescence, granulomas in the histology, and the role of genetic factors were found, suggesting that our case is CGD-like disorder, manifested in an adult. Dialysable leukocyte extract (DLE) therapy, complemented with fresh normal plasma, resulted in a striking clinical improvement and there was an increase in the in vitro PMNL intracellular killing activity, too. Although it is generally accepted that DLE derives from monocytes and lymphocytes, it is possible that DLE is a family of DNA-oligopeptide molecules, including factors derived from PMNLs which are capable of influencing PMNL function, transferring information from normal cells. Our results also suggest that it would be worth trying DLE in patients with classic CGD.

[89]

Wilson GB. Poindexter C. Fort JD. Ludden KD. **De novo initiation of specific cell-mediated immune responsiveness in chickens by transfer factor (specific immunity inducer) obtained from bovine colostrum and milk.** Acta Virologica. 32(1):6-18, 1988.

Transfer factors (TF) were prepared from colostrum and milk of bovines previously immunized with antigens obtained from Coccidioides immitis, infectious bovine rhinotracheitis virus, or from the viral agents responsible for avian Newcastle disease, laryngotracheitis disease or infectious bursal disease. The ability of bovine TF to transfer specific cell-mediated immune responsiveness to a markedly xenogenic species was studied using specific pathogen free (SPF) and standard commercial (SC) chickens as model recipients. Cell-mediated immune responsiveness was documented using one or more of the following for each antigen (organism) studied: (a) an in vitro chicken leukocyte (heterophil) migration inhibition assay; (b) delayed-wattle reactivity; or (c) protection from clinical disease. Chicken TFs obtained from spleens of immune donors were evaluated in parallel to bovine TF's in selected comparative studies. Bovine TF also referred to as specific immunity inducer (SII), and chicken TF were found to initiate antigen-specific cell-mediated immunity de novo in previously non-immune SPF chickens as well as in SC chickens despite the presence of maternally acquired humoral antibody which may serve as a "barrier" to immunization of SC chickens when commercially available vaccines are administered by parenteral routes. Bovine TF's specific for laryngotracheitis virus or infectious bursal disease virus afforded protection equal to that found for commercially available vaccines. Bovine TF's action was rapid (less than a day) and of relatively long duration at least 35 days.

[90]

Miller LL. Spitler LE. Allen RE. Minor DR. Paul M. A **randomized, double-blind, placebo-controlled trial of transfer factor as adjuvant therapy for malignant melanoma.** Cancer. 61(8):1543-9, 1988.

One hundred and sixty-eight evaluable patients participated in a randomized, double-blind study of transfer factor (TF) versus placebo as surgical adjuvant therapy of Stage I and Stage II malignant melanoma. Eighty-five patients received TF prepared from the leukocytes of healthy volunteer donors; eighty-three participants received placebo. Therapy was initiated within 90 days of resection of all evident tumor and continued until 2 years of disease-free survival or the occurrence of unresectable dissemination of melanoma. Known prognostic variables were similarly distributed in the treatment and control groups, documenting the randomization efficacy. Three endpoints were analyzed: disease-free interval, time to Stage III metastasis, and survival. After a median follow-up period of 24.75 months, there was a trend in favor of the placebo group with regard to all three endpoints and this was significant (P less than or equal to 0.05) for time to Stage III metastasis. These findings indicate that TF is not effective as surgical adjuvant therapy of malignant melanoma.

[91]

Pogodina VV. Levina LS. Perepechkina NP. Mats AN. **The effect of preparations of specific and nonspecific transfer-factor on the course of experimental tick-borne encephalitis.** Voprosy Virusologii. 34(6):689-94, 1989.

Syrian hamsters subcutaneously inoculated with tick-borne encephalitis (TBE) virus were given transfer-factor (TF) preparations derived by different methods. The preparation of specific TF was obtained from the blood leukocytes of TBE convalescents. The nonspecific TF preparations were made of the lymphocytes of the tonsils removed from children with chronic tonsillitis outside the TBE focus. The effect of the TF preparations depended on the TBE virus strain and dose, TF preparation dosage schedule and characteristics. The specific TF preparations stimulated the development of acute fatal TBE after 3 injections at intervals of 0, 48 and 96 hours postinoculation with the virus. The preparations of nonspecific TF potentiate the infection after preliminary (24 hours) and simultaneous inoculation of the virus, producing transformation of asymptomatic infection to subacute TBE or exacerbation of the subacute process. A significant inhibition of TBE virus reproduction in spleen and brain tissues is observed after inoculation of a nonspecific TF F150 preparation 72 hours after virus inoculation, that is at the time when the virus has been already localized in the central nervous system. The results of the study indicate that the protective effect of TF is mainly associated with nonspecific immunopharmacological activity of the preparations.

[92]

Iseki M. Aoyama T. Koizumi Y. Ojima T. Murase Y. Osano M. **Effects of transfer factor on chronic hepatitis B in childhood.** Kansenshogaku Zasshi - Journal of the Japanese Association for Infectious Diseases. 63(12):1329-32, 1989.

Nine children, 1 to 13 years of age, with HBeAg positive chronic hepatitis B received transfer factor (T.F.) monotherapy for 3 to 17 months, and were monitored by check-ups every six months from serum HBeAg, anti-

HBe and GPT. In 12 months, 4 subjects became HBeAg negative and had normal serum GPT. In 22 to 48 months, 6 of the nine subjects had negative HBeAg and normal GPT, 2 had positive HBeAg and high GPT values. The remaining 1 subject who was observed for six months after T.F. therapy remained HBeAg positive with a high GPT values. No side effects were observed. These preliminary observations may indicate beneficial effects of T.F. on the natural course of chronic hepatitis B in childhood, though the ultimate effects awaits longer and well controlled clinical trials.

[93]

Vezendi S. Schroder I. **Transfer factor therapy of thoracic sarcoidosis.** Allergologia et Immunopathologia. 17(1):35-7, 1989.

The authors repeatedly treated 59 patients with thoracic sarcoidosis with transfer factor (TF) since 1976. They utilized this therapy with TF from human tonsil lymphocyte (TFh) on account of the ineffectiveness of the corticosteroid treatment, because of the side effects of the corticosteroids, and as primary TF therapy, and to test an animal TF preparation from pig tonsil lymphocytes (TFp). In their observations only fraction II of the dialysable leukocyte extract was sufficient. Differences in the effectiveness between TFh and TFp do not exist on the whole. Our conclusion is that TF can stimulate the immunosystem of the patients, and can be an important mode of treatment. The mode of action is not clear.

[94]

Neequaye J. Viza D. Pizza G. Levine PH. De Vinci C. Ablashi DV. Biggar RJ. Nkrumah FK. **Specific transfer factor with activity against Epstein-Barr virus reduces late relapse in endemic Burkitt's lymphoma.** Anticancer Research. 10(5A):1183-7, 1990.

Twenty-seven children with abdominal Burkitt's lymphoma (stage III), who had achieved complete remission, were entered into a prospective controlled trial of adjunct treatment with Epstein-Barr virus (EBV)-specific transfer factor (TF). Two patients treated with TF and 2 controls relapsed early (less than or equal to 12 weeks). Two out of 12 TF-treated patients and 5 out of 11 controls subsequently suffered relapses. Time to first late relapse was longer among TF-treated patients (p = 0.08), and no late relapse occurred while a patient was receiving TF treatment. Thus it seems that specific TF might be useful in the management of endemic Burkitt's lymphoma and also in the treatment of other virus-associated cancers and diseases.

[95]

McMeeking A. Borkowsky W. Klesius PH. Bonk S. Holzman RS. Lawrence HS. **A controlled trial of bovine dialyzable leukocyte extract for cryptosporidiosis in patients with AIDS**. Journal of Infectious Diseases. 161(1):108-12, 1990.

Cryptosporidial infection causes severe diarrheal disease in patients with AIDS. Fourteen patients with AIDS and symptomatic cryptosporidiosis were treated with a specific bovine dialyzable leukocyte extract (immune DLE) prepared from lymph node lymphocytes of calves immunized with cryptosporidia or a nonspecific (nonimmune) DLE prepared from nonimmunized calves. Six of 7 patients given immune DLE gained weight and had a decrease in bowel movement frequency, with eradication of oocysts from stool in 5 patients. Six of 7 patients given nonimmune DLE showed no decrease in bowel movement and 4, no clearing of oocytes from stool; 5 continued to lose weight. Subsequently, 5 of these 7 were treated with immune DLE; 4 had a decrease in bowel movement frequency and significant weight gain, with eradication of oocytes from stool in 2 patients. Immune DLE produces sustained symptomatic improvement in patients with AIDS and active cryptosporidiosis, but lack of an appropriate cryptosporidial antigen allows only postulation that an augmentation of cellular immunity to Cryptosporidium parvum induced by immune DLE resulted in the microbiologic and clinical improvement observed.

[96]

Sumiyama K. Kobayashi M. Miyashiro E. Koike M. **Combination therapy with transfer factor and high dose stronger neo-minophagen C in chronic hepatitis B in children (HBe Ag positive)**. Acta Paediatrica Japonica. 33(3):327-34, 1991.

This study mainly describes the efficacy of the combination therapy with Transfer Factor (TF) and high dose Stronger Neo-Minophagen C (SNMC) for HBV carrier children with HBe Ag positive chronic hepatitis. There were 12 patients, 10 males and 2 females aged from 7 months to 14 years 8 months. Liver biopsy was done in 11 patients, and the histopathological findings of the liver were chronic active hepatitis (8 cases) and chronic inactive hepatitis (3 cases). In 6 of 8 patients, HBe-Ag became negative (75%) within 18 weeks (mean 8 weeks) after the initiation of the combination therapy with TF and SNMC (HBe-seronegative), and 4 of these 8 patients (50%) became anti-HBe positive within 29 weeks (mean 15 weeks) (HBe-seroconversion). These results suggest that combination therapy with TF and high dose SNMC may be beneficial in the treatment of chronic hepatitis B in children.

[97]

Qi HY. Wan ZF. Su CZ. **Isolation and purification of HSV-1 specific transfer factor produced by HSV-1 immunized goat leukocyte dialysate**. Acta Virologica. 36(3):231-8, 1992.

A herpes simplex virus type 1 (HSV-1)-specific transfer factor (TF), was separated and purified from the leukocyte dialysate of goats immunized with HSV-1 using affinity chromatography on antigen-sorbent and reversed phase high performance liquid chromatography (RP-HPLC). The antigen-specific activities of the starting dialysate and the isolated TF component (s) were examined by 51Cr-labelled leukocyte adherence inhibition (51Cr LAI) assay. The analytical hydrophobic interaction HPLC (HI-HPLC) and isoelectric focusing (IEF) techniques were employed to evaluate the purity and the isoelectric point (PI) of isolated TF component(s). The experiments provided a two-step procedure for purifying the TF material from the starting dialysate. It seems that the purified active TF component (PTFC) was specific for HSV-1. The specific PTFC activity was increased 10,000-fold as compared with the activity of the dialysate. The active moiety appeared as a single band in the IEF gel as demonstrated by silver staining; it was hydrophilic and its PI was pH 4.48.

[98]

Xu WM. **Determination of antigen-dependent activity of human lung cancer transfer factor by H3-leucine leucine leukocyte adherence inhibition assay.** [Chinese] Chung-Hua Chung Liu Tsa Chih [Chinese Journal of Oncology]. 14(2):116-8, 1992.

This report is to demonstrate the antigen-dependent activity of human lung cancer transfer factor (Sp-TF). Sp-TFM was prepared from spleen of mice immunized with the human lung cancer cell line A549. [3H]-leu leukocyte adherence inhibition assay ([3H]-leu-LAI) was modified to identify activity of Sp-TFM. Leukocytes obtained from non-immunized mice were divided into eight groups as follows: 1. Control without TF or antigen; 2. Sp-TFM and antigen of cell line A549 (A549 Ag); 3. Sp-TFM alone; 4. Sp-TFM and ascitic tumor cell H22 antigen of mice (H22Ag); 5. Sp-TFM and antigen of human gastric cancer cell (HGCCAg); 6. Sp-TFM and antigen of human normal lung tissue (NLTAg); 7. Nor special TF of mice (N-TFM) and A549Ag; 8. A549Ag alone. When normal leukocytes were incubated with Sp-TFM and A549 antigen, the leukocytes adherence inhibition index (LAII) was significantly higher than those of the other groups. The different LAII of Sp-TFM to A549Ag and other experimental groups were highly significant (P less than 0.001). The results demonstrated that Sp-TFM could transfer specific cell mediated immunity to non-immune leukocytes. The TF prepared from spleen of goat immunized with antigen from lung cancer of patients (Sp-TFG) showed antigen specific activity as well as Sp-TFM.

[99]

Qi HY. Wan ZF. Su CZ. **Chemical characterization of the purified component of specific transfer factor in the leukocyte dialysates from HSV-1 immunized goats.** Acta Virologica. 36(3):239-44, 1992.

he chemical characterization of the purified component responsible for HSV-1 specific transfer factor activity (PTFC) by high resolution analytical methods was performed. PTFC had a molecular weight of 6,000 dalton by the size-exclusion HPLC analysis; it showed a marked UV-absorbance spot at 254 nm and a fluorescent spot at 366 nm on the thin-layer plate by thin-layer chromatography which spots coincided at the same place of the plate. The amino acid composition and sequencing analyses showed that PTFC consisted of at least twelve different amino acids, but the amino acid sequence could not be determined. The combined results indicate that PTFC is a compound with a molecular weight of 6,000 dalton, composed of peptide and nucleotide-like material. The peptide is rich in aspartic acid and its N-terminal end may be blocked.

[100]

Mikula I. Pistl J. Rosocha J. **Dialyzable leukocyte extract used in the prevention of Salmonella infection in calves.** Veterinary Immunology & Immunopathology. 32(1-2):113-24, 1992.

The protective effect of dialyzable leukocyte extract (DLE) was investigated in the experimental model of Salmonella infection in calves. DLE was obtained from the lymphatic nodes and spleens of fattening bulls immunized with whole-cell Salmonella vaccine (designated DLEs-im), from the same organs of calves immunized and subsequently infected with Salmonella typhimurium (DLEs-inf), and from non-immunized fattening bulls (DLEn). Three doses of DLEs-inf and DLEs-im applied intravenously at 3-day intervals induced protection in all calves against infection. There were statistically significant differences in the immunological, clinical and microbio-logical parameters. Three doses of DLEs-inf injected intramuscularly at 3-day intervals provided a protective effect; however, one calf died. The intravenous application of DLEn induced low protection against experimental Salmonella infection and two calves died. The results indicate that the preparation of antigen-specific DLE may be possible via immunization of fattening bulls.

[101]

Whyte RI. Schork MA. Sloan H. Orringer MB. Kirsh MM. **Adjuvant treatment using transfer factor for bronchogenic carcinoma: long-term follow-up.** Annals of Thoracic Surgery. 53(3):391-6, 1992.

Transfer factor, a dialyzable lymphocyte extract that may act as an immune stimulator by transferring antigen-specific immunity between genetically dissimilar individuals, was administered in a prospective, randomized study to patients with non-small cell bronchogenic carcinoma. Between 1976 and 1982, 63 patients who underwent pulmonary resection, mediastinal lymph node dissection, and, when indicated by the presence of mediastinal lymph node involvement, mediastinal irradiation were randomized into two groups. Group 1 (n = 28) received 1 mL of pooled transfer factor at 3-month intervals after operation; group 2 (n = 35) served as controls and received saline solution. There were no statistically significant differences between the two groups with respect to age, sex, tumor histology, stage of disease, or extent of resection. One patient was lost to follow-up at 96 months; follow-up was complete in all others through July 1990. In patients receiving transfer factor, the 2-, 5-, and 10-year survival rates were 82%, 64%, and 43% respectively, whereas in controls they were 63%, 43%, and 23%. Survival in patients receiving transfer factor was consistently better than in those receiving placebo. Furthermore, survival in patients receiving transfer factor was greater at all stages of disease for both adenocarcinoma and squamous cell carcinoma. Although these long-term results were not statistically significant using survival analysis with covariates (p = 0.08), they confirm our previously reported short-term findings suggesting that administration of transfer factor, either through nonspecific immune stimulation, enhancement of cell-mediated immunity, or an as yet undefined mechanism, can improve survival in patients with bronchogenic carcinoma.

[102]

Mrazova A. Mraz J. **Transfer factor and its signification for practice.** Sbornik Vedeckych Praci Lekarske Fakulty Karlovy Univerzity V Hradci Kralove. 36(3):117-37, 1993.

In the study literary data are given together with our own experience with the immunomodulation effects of Transfer Factor (TF) Sevac. The application of 3-5 ampulles of TF leads not only to E rosettes but even to a separate subpopulations of T lymphocytes increase. The results obtained in 51 patients with GIT and renal cells carcinoma were statistically evaluated. About 80% of the patients experienced an improvement of subjective conditions during the treatment. Objectively supported adjustment of laboratory indices was found in 83-88% of the parameters evaluated. Also the absolute numbers of CD4+ cells in 10(9)/1 increased (at p < 0.001) together with CD3+ and

CD8+ (p < 0.01). A significant correlation between separate subpopulations of T lymphocytes and B lymphocytes was proved in the original mode. From our results it is obvious that the TF Sevac application and further observing of its immunomodulation effect will be the object of interest of the immunologists of general practice and clinical research even in spite of some lacks in its characteristics.

[103]

Pen GY. **Effect of hepatocellular carcinoma-specific transfer factor (HCC-S-TF) on IL-2 activity and IL-2R expression**. [Chinese] Chung-Hua Chung Liu Tsa Chih [Chinese Journal of Oncology]. 15(6):435-7, 1993.

HCC specific transfer factor (S-TF) was extracted from lymphoid tissues of goats immunized with HCC cell suspension. The effect of the S-TF on IL-2 activity and IL-2R expression was observed in vitro. The results showed that IL-2 activity and IL-2R expression in HCC patients but not in normal subjects could be increased by the S-TF. The IL-2 activities and IL-2R expressions in both normal subjects and patients with HCC could not be increased by normal transfer factor (N-TF). This may be one of the anti-tumor mechanisms of S-TF. It suggests that S-TF may be better than N-TF in immunotherapy of human tumors.

[104]

Valdes Sanchez AF. Martin Rodriguez OL. Lastra Alfonso G. **Treatment of extrinsic bronchial asthma with transfer factor.** [Spanish]Revista Alergia Mexico. 40(5):124-31, 1993.

A group of 90 external asthmatics with cellular immunodeficiency or not was studied and treated during 10 months with transfer factor or double blind placebo. Total immunoglobulin serum studies (A, G, M and E), spontaneous rosette and intradermal tests, were made a month before the treatment's beginning and a month after the ending of the treatment. The patients were clinically evaluated every day in accordance to the intensity and the frequency of their crisis and with the immunological point of view of the tests made. There was not significant differences between the study groups treated with the transfer factor or not. Adverse reactions were not noticed.

[105]

Fernandez, O. Diaz, N. Morales, E. Toledo, J. Hernandez, E. Rojas, S. Madriz, X. Lopez Saura, P. **Effect of transfer factor on myelosuppression and related morbidity induced by chemotherapy in acute leukaemias.** British Journal of Haematology. 84(3):423-7, 1993.

The aim of this study is to determine the safety and efficacy of Transfer Factor (TF) in accelerating the haematopoietic recovery in patients with acute leukaemias (AL), following intensive therapy to induce remission of the disease. Twenty-two patients with different types of AL (16 AML, three BC-CML and three ALL) were studied. The patients were divided in two groups. Group 1 (eight AML, two BC-CML and one ALL) received, after myelosuppression induced by chemotherapy, TF (1 unit daily, subcutaneous) until leucocyte count was > 2.5 x 10(9)/l and platelet count > 80 x 10(9)/l. Group 2 was considered the control group and did not receive TF. Treatment with TF accelerated the recovery of neutrophils, leucocytes, platelets (P < 0.001) and haemoglobin (P < 0.01). As a logical consequence, incidence and severity of infection and haemorrhage were lesser in the TF group than in the control group. There was no evidence that TF accelerated the re-growth of leukaemic cells. It seems that TF is safe in AL, accelerating haematopoietic recovery. However, it should be used with caution until results of additional trials become available.

[106]

Ferrer-Argote VE. Romero-Cabello R. Hernandez-Mendoza L. Arista-Viveros A. Rojo-Medina J. Balseca-Olivera F. Fierro M. Gonzalez-Constandse R. **Successful treatment of severe complicated measles with non-specific transfer factor.** In Vivo. 8(4):555-7, 1994.

Severe complicated measles has a high mortality rate and no specific treatment. Ten patients with complicated measles - 9 infants with respiratory failure and a 15 year old boy with encephalitis - received immunotherapy with Non-specific Transfer Factor (NTF). The patients had variable degrees of undernourishment and were severely ill when immunotherapy was started. 8/9 cases with respiratory failure were cured. One died of bronchoaspiration while recovering from the measles. The case with encephalitis showed no neurological sequelae two weeks after receiving the last dose of NTF. Treatment of complicated measles with NTF in these patients seemed very effective and deserves further trial.

[107]

Pizza G. Meduri R. De Vinci C. Scorolli L. Viza D. **Transfer factor prevents relapses in herpes keratitis patients: a pilot study.** Biotherapy. 8(1):63-8, 1994.

Transfer Factor is a dialysable moiety obtained from immune lymphocytes. It has been successfully used for the treatment of several viral infections including labial and genital herpes. In the present study, thirty-three patients with low immune response to HSV antigens and suffering from herpes ocular infections were orally treated with HSV-specific transfer factor (TF). Their relapse index was reduced from 20.1 before treatment to 0.51 after TF administration, with only 6/33 patients relapsing. Although this is not a placebo-controlled-randomized study, the results suggest that TF specific for HSV antigens may be efficacious for preventing relapses of ocular herpes infections as has been the case with genital and labial localisations.

[108]

Stancikova M. Rovensky J. Pekarek J. Orvisky E. Blazickova S. Cech K. **Influence of various forms of dialyzable leukocyte extracts on rat adjuvant arthritis.** Archivum Immunologiae et Therapiae Experimentalis. 42(4):295-9, 1994.

Adjuvant-induced arthritis in rats is a chronic inflammatory disease, widely used as an animal model for rheumatoid arthritis. In our study the effect of various fractions of dialyzable leukocyte extract (DLE): DLE I-molecular weight below 10 kDa (commercial preparation), DLE II-molecular weight below 5 kDa (suppressor fraction), DLE III-molecular weight 5-10 kDa on rat adjuvant-induced arthritis was studied. The adjuvant arthritic (AA) rats were treated with DLE fractions i.p. in solutions containing an active substance isolated from 12.5 x 10(6) and 6.25 x 10(6) leukocytes from day 1 (adjuvant injected) through day 18, every second day (total 9 times). Various markers of inflammation, immune function and joint destruction were evaluated: hindpaw volume, serum hyaluronic acid, serum albumin and biopterin in urine. All these markers showed a significant improvement after using fraction DLE II in comparison with AA controls. Fractions DLE I and DLE III influenced only some markers of inflammation and immune function. Our results demonstrated a therapeutical effect of fraction DLE II on rat adjuvant-induced arthritis.

[109]

Estrada-Parra S. Chavez-Sanchez R. Ondarza-Aguilera R. Correa-Meza B. Serrano-Miranda E. Monges-Nicolau A. Calva-Pellicer C. **Immunotherapy with transfer factor of recurrent herpes simplex type I.**
Archives of Medical Research. 26 Spec No:S87-92, 1995.

This clinical trial of Transfer Factor, an immunomodulator, in the treatment of herpes simplex type I, proved this agent to be more effective as regards duration of acute phase recurrences as well as the frequency of the reappearance of relapses of this disease. The evaluation was made in 20 patients whose disease had been treated before with other therapeutic agents (including acyclovir) which permitted them to be their own controls for the comparative data obtained and submitted to statistical analysis of the two parameters mentioned, duration of the acute phase and frequency of relapses. Patients with compromised cellular immunity or with any additional disease were excluded from the study. Transfer factor, one unit, was administered subcutaneously daily for 3 to 4 days during the acute phase of the disease, and subsequently at 15-day intervals for the first 6 months; followed by a continuation of monthly injections until the termination of the study period. In six of the 20 patients there was a recurrence of the disease while receiving maintenance dosages of TF. These patients were again given the full initial dosage schedule and reinstated again with the maintenance dosage. In the initial eight patients, an immune status profile was obtained, and all results were found to be in the normal range. This was considered sufficient evidence that the criteria for the selection of patients excluded any with detectable variations in the profile of the immune status, and it was decided to eliminate this as a prerequisite for participating in the study. The results showed an important improvement in the response to transfer factor immune modulation therapy. A statistically significant reduction in the frequency of recurrences within a one month period, the Student t test gave a $p = 0.0001$ in TF treated patients. The average duration in days of the acute phase also showed an important difference in favor of the TF treatment. The U Mann-Whitney test gave a $p = 0.0005$. These results suggest that, at present, TF may be considered the therapeutic agent of choice in the treatment of herpes simplex type 1 disease.

[110]

Pizza G. Viza D. De Vinci C. Palareti A. Cuzzocrea D. Fornarola V. Baricordi R. **Orally administered HSV-specific transfer factor (TF) prevents genital or labial herpes relapses**. Biotherapy. 9(1-3):67-72, 1996.

Forty-four patients suffering from genital (22) and labial (22) herpes were orally treated with HSV-1/2-specific transfer factor (TF). TF was obtained by in vitro replication of a HSV-1/2-specific bovine dialysable lymphocyte extract. Treatment was administered bi-weekly the first 2 weeks, and then weekly for 6 months, most patients received 2-3 courses. The total observation period for all patients before treatment was 26,660 days, with 544 relapses, and a relapse index of 61.2, whereas the cumulative observation period during and after treatment was 16,945 days, with a total of 121 relapsing episodes and a cumulative RI of 21.4 ($P < 0.0001$). Results were equally significant when the 2 groups of patients (labial and genital) were considered separately. These observations confirm previous results obtained with bovine HSV-specific TF, and warrant further studies to establish HSV-specific TF as a choice of treatment for preventing herpes recurrences.

[111]

Byston J. Cech K. Pekarek J. Jilkova J. **Effect of anti-herpes specific transfer factor.** Biotherapy. 9(1-3):73-5, 1996.

Using a blood cell separator, lymphocytes were collected from otherwise healthy convalescents suffering from herpetic infections. A specific anti-herpes dialysate (AH-DLE) was prepared from the lymphocytes, using standard procedures. Patients with recurrent herpetic infections were treated with a single dose of the dialysate, at the initial signs of herpetic infection (group A), with two doses (group B) or with three doses (group C). A total number of 37 patients (29 women, 8 men, age range 15-73 years) were treated. No improvement was observed in 7 patients (18.9%), whilst 7 patients did not manifest any exacerbation of their herpetic infection in the course of the one-year follow-up. The remaining 62.2% of the patients showed a marked improvement: decrease of the frequency and/or duration or relapses. Before AH-DLE administration, the mean number of herpes relapses in this group of patients was 12 p.a.. After therapy, the number of relapses decreased to 3.5 p.a.. No statistically significant difference was observed between groups A and B. The least favourable results were registered in group C. However, this group included 6 female patients extremely resistant to the previously therapeutic attempts, including inosiplex, non-specific DLE or acyclovir. Thus, even in this group, the therapy was successful in 50% of the patients.

[112]

Ablashi DV. Levine PH. De Vinci C. Whitman JE Jr. Pizza G. Viza D. **Use of anti HHV-6 transfer factor for the treatment of two patients with chronic fatigue syndrome (CFS). Two case reports**. Biotherapy. 9(1-3):81-6, 1996.

Specific Human Herpes virus-6 (HHV-6) transfer factor (TF) preparation, administered to two chronic fatigue syndrome patients, inhibited the HHV-6 infection. Prior to treatment, both patients exhibited an activated HHV-6 infection. TF treatment significantly improved the clinical manifestations of CFS in one patient who resumed normal duties within weeks, whereas no clinical improvement was observed in the second patient. It is concluded that HHV-6 specific TF may be of significant value in controlling HHV-6 infection and related illnesses.

[113]

De Vinci C. Levine PH. Pizza G. Fudenberg HH. Orens P. Pearson G. Viza D. **Lessons from a pilot study of transfer factor in chronic fatigue syndrome.** Biotherapy. 9(1-3):87-90, 1996.

Transfer Factor (TF) was used in a placebo controlled pilot study of 20 patients with chronic fatigue syndrome (CFS). Efficacy of the treatment was evaluated by clinical monitoring and testing for antibodies to Epstein-Barr virus (EBV) and human herpes virus-6 (HHV-6). Of the 20 patients in the placebo-controlled trial, improvement was observed in 12 patients, generally within 3-6 weeks of beginning treatment. Herpes virus serology seldom correlated with clinical response. This study provided experience with oral TF, useful in designing a larger placebo-controlled clinical trial.

[114]

Hana I. Vrubel J. Pekarek J. Cech K. **The influence of age on transfer factor treatment of cellular immunodeficiency, chronic fatigue syndrome and/or chronic viral infections.** Biotherapy. 9(1-3):91-5, 1996.

A group of 222 patients suffering from cellular immunodeficiency (CID), frequently combined with chronic fatigue syndrome (CFS) and/or chronic viral infections by Epstein-Barr virus (EBV) and/or cytomegalovirus (CMV), were immunologically investigated and treated with transfer factor (TF). The age range was 17-77 years. In order to elucidate the influence of aging on the course of the disease and on treatment, 3 subgroups were formed: 17-43 years, 44-53 years, and 54-77 years. Six injections of Immodin (commercial preparation of TF by SEVAC, Prague) were given in the course of 8 weeks. When active viral infection was present, IgG injections and vitamins were added. Immunological investigation was performed before the start of therapy, and subsequently according to need, but not later than after 3 months. The percentages of failures to improve clinical status of patients were in the individual subgroups, respectively: 10.6%, 11.5% and 28.9%. The influence of increasing age on the percentage of failures to normalize low numbers of T cells was very evident: 10.6%, 21.2% and 59.6%. In individuals uneffected by therapy, persistent absolute lymphocyte numbers below 1,200 cells were found in 23.1%, 54.5% and 89.3% in the oldest group. Statistical analysis by Pearson's Chi-square test, and the test for linear trend proved that the differences among the individual age groups were significant. Neither sex, nor other factors seemed to influence the results. The results of this pilot study show that age substantially influences the failure rate of CID treatment using TF. In older people, it is easier to improve the clinical condition than CID: this may be related to the diminished number of lymphocytes, however, a placebo effect cannot be totally excluded.

[115]

Pizza G. De Vinci C. Fornarola V. Palareti A. Baricordi O. Viza D. **In vitro studies during long-term oral administration of specific transfer factor.** Biotherapy. 9(1-3):175-85, 1996.

153 patients suffering from recurrent pathologies, i.e. viral infections (keratitis, keratouveitis, genital and labial herpes) uveitis, cystitis, and candidiasis were treated with in vitro produced transfer factor (TF) specific for HSV-1/2, CMV and Candida albicans. The cell-mediated immunity of seropositive patients to HSV-1/2 and/or CMV viruses was assessed using the leucocyte migration inhibition test (LMT) and lymphocyte stimulation test (LST) in

presence of the corresponding antigens, and the frequency of positive tests before, during and after TF administration was studied. The data were stratified per type of test, antigen and the recipients' pathology, and statistically evaluated. For the LMT, a total of 960 tests were carried out for each antigen dilution, 3 different antigen dilutions were used per test. 240/960 tests (25.4%) were found positive during non-treatment or treatment with unspecific TF, whereas 147/346 tests (42.5%) were found positive when the antigen corresponding to the specificity of the TF administered to the patient was used ($P < 0.001$). When the data were stratified following pathology, a significant increased incidence of positive tests during specific treatment was also observed ($0.0001 < P < 0.05$). In the LST (1174 tests), a significant increase of thymidine uptake was observed in the absence of antigen (control cultures), during treatment with both specific and unspecific TF, but also in the presence of antigen and/or autologous serum during specific TF administration ($P < 0.0001$). TF administration also significantly increased the soluble HLA class I antigens level in 40 patients studied to this effect.

[116]

Masi M. De Vinci C. Baricordi OR. **Transfer factor in chronic mucocutaneous candidiasis.** Biotherapy. 9(1-3):97-103, 1996.

Fifteen patients suffering from chronic mucocutaneous candidiasis were treated with an in vitro produced TF specific for Candida albicans antigens and/or with TF extracted from pooled buffy coats of blood donors. CMI of the patients was assessed using the LMT and the LST in presence of candidine. The aim of the study was the clinical evaluation of TF treatment and the incidence of positive tests before, during, and after therapy. Immunological data were matched using the Chi square test. 87 LMT were performed for each antigen dose and at the dilution of 1/50, 58.9% (33/56) tests were positive during non-treatment or non-specific TF treatment. On the contrary 83.9% (26/31) were positive during specific TF treatment ($P < 0.05$). In the LST, a significant decrease of thymidine uptake in the control cultures in presence of autologous or AB serum was observed when patients were matched according to non-treatment, and both non specific ($P < 0.05$) and specific TF treatment ($P < 0.01$). Only during specific TF treatment was a significant increase of reactivity against the Candida antigen at the highest concentration noticed, when compared with the period of non specific treatment ($P < 0.01$). Clinical observations were encouraging: all but one patient experienced significant improvement during treatment with specific TF. These data confirm that orally administered specific TF, extracted from induced lymphoblastoid cell-lines, increases the incidence of reactivity against Candida antigens in the LMT. LST reactivity appeared not significantly increased with respect to the periods of non treatment, but was significantly increased when it was compared to the non-specific TF treatment periods. At the same time, a clinical improvement was noticed.

[117]

Prasad U. bin Jalaludin MA. Rajadurai P. Pizza G. De Vinci C. Viza D. Levine PH. **Transfer factor with anti-EBV activity as an adjuvant therapy for nasopharyngeal carcinoma: a pilot study**. Biotherapy. 9(1-3):109-15, 1996.

Overall survival of nasopharyngeal carcinoma (NPC) at UICC stage IV still remains unsatisfactory even with combination chemotherapy (CT) and radio-therapy (RT). In view of the association of reactivation of Epstein-Barr virus (EBV) with the development and recurrence of NPC, immunotherapy in the form of transfer factor (TF) with specific activity against EBV (TF-B1) was suggested as an adjuvant to a combination of CT and RT in order to improve survival. In the present study, 6 UICC stage IV patients received TF-B1 and another 6 patients matched for disease stage were given TF prepared from peripheral blood leucocytes (TF-PBL). Results were compared with another 18 patients matched by age, sex, and stage of disease who received standard therapy without TF during the same period (C group). After a median follow up of 47.5 months, the survival for the TF-B1 group was found to be significantly better (P = < 0.05) than the PBL and C group. While the 8 patients with distant metastasis (DM), not treated with TF-B1 (6 in the control and 2 in the PBL group), died due to progressive disease (average survival being 14.3 months), both patients with DM in the TF-B1 group had complete remission: one died of tuberculosis after surviving for 3.5 years and another is still alive, disease free, after 4.2 years. Although the series involved a small number of cases, the apparent effect of adjuvant immunotherapy in the form of TF with anti-EBV activity is of considerable interest.

[118]

Pilotti V. Mastrorilli M. Pizza G. De Vinci C. Busutti L. Palareti A. Gozzetti G. Cavallari A. **Transfer factor as an adjuvant to non-small cell lung** cancer (NSCLC) therapy. Biotherapy. 9(1-3):117-21, 1996.

The rationale for using transfer factor (TF) in lung cancer patients is that the possibility of improving their cell-mediated immunity to tumour associated antigens (TAA) may improve their survival. From Jan 1984 to Jan 1995, 99 non-small cell lung cancer (NSCLC) resected patients were monthly treated with TF, extracted from the lymphocytes of blood bank donors. In the same period, 257 NSCLC resected patients were considered as non-treated controls. The survival rates of the TF treated group appear significantly improved both for patients in stages 3a and 3b, and patients with histological subtype "large cell carcinoma" (P < 0.02). Survival of TF treated patients is also significantly higher (P < 0.02) for patients with lymph node involvement (N2 disease). The results of this study suggest that the administration of TF to NSCLC resected patients may improve survival.

[119]

Pizza G. De Vinci C. Cuzzocrea D. Menniti D. Aiello E. Maver P. Corrado G. Romagnoli P. Dragoni E. LoConte G. Riolo U. Palareti A. Zucchelli P. Fornarola V. Viza D. **A preliminary report on the use of transfer factor for treating stage D3 hormone-unresponsive metastatic prostate cancer.** Biotherapy. 9(1-3):123-32, 1996.

As conventional treatments are unsuccessful, the survival rate of stage D3 prostate cancer patients is poor. Reports have suggested the existence of humoral and cell-mediated immunity (CMI) against prostate cancer tumour-associated antigens (TAA). These observations prompted us to treat stage D3 prostate cancer patients with an in vitro produced transfer factor (TF) able to transfer, in vitro and in vivo, CMI against bladder and prostate TAA. Fifty patients entered this study and received one intramuscular injection of 2-5 units of specific TF monthly. Follow-up, ranging from 1 to 9 years, showed that complete remission was achieved in 2 patients, partial remission in 6, and no progression of metastatic disease in 14. The median survival was 126 weeks, higher than the survival rates reported in the literature for patients of the same stage.

[120]

De Vinci C. Pizza G. Cuzzocrea D. Menniti D. Aiello E. Maver P. Corrado G. Romagnoli P. Dragoni E. LoConte G. Riolo U. Masi M. Severini G. Fornarola V. Viza D. **Use of transfer factor for the treatment of recurrent non-bacterial female cystitis (NBRC): a preliminary report.** Biotherapy. 9(1-3):133-8, 1996.

Results of conventional treatment of female non-bacterial recurrent cystitis (NBRC) are discouraging. Most patients show an unexpected high incidence of vaginal candidiasis, while their cell mediated immunity to Herpes simplex viruses (HSV) and Candida antigens seems impaired, and it is known that the persistence of mucocutaneous chronic candidiasis is mainly due to a selective defect of CMI to Candida antigens. Twenty nine women suffering of NBRC, and in whom previous treatment with antibiotics and non-steroid anti-inflammatory drugs was unsuccessful, underwent oral transfer factor (TF) therapy. TF specific to Candida and/or to HSV was administered bi-weekly for the first 2 weeks, and then once a week for the following 6 months. No side effects were observed during treatment. The total observation period of our cohort was 24379 days with 353 episodes of cystitis recorded and a cumulative relapse index (RI) of 43. The observation period during and after treatment was 13920 days with 108 relapses and a cumulative RI of 23 (P < 0.0001). It, thus, seems that specific TF may be capable of controlling NBRC and alleviate the symptoms.

[121]

Meduri R. Campos E. Scorolli L. De Vinci C. Pizza G. Viza D. **Efficacy of transfer factor in treating patients with recurrent ocular herpes infections.** Biotherapy. 9(1-3):61-6, 1996.

Recurrent ocular herpes is an insoluble problem for the clinician. As cellular immunity plays an important role in controlling herpes relapses, and other studies have shown the efficacy of HSV-specific transfer factor (TF) for the treatment of herpes patients, an open clinical trial was undertaken in 134 patients (71 keratitis, 29 kerato-uveitis, 34 uveitis) suffering from recurrent ocular herpetic infections. The mean duration of the treatment was 358 days, and the entire follow-up period 189,121 before, and 64,062 days after TF treatment. The cell-mediated immune response to the viral antigens, evaluated by the lymphocyte stimulation test (LST) and the leucocyte migration test (LMT) (P < 0.001), was significantly increased by the TF treatment. The total number of relapses was decreased significantly during/after TF treatment, dropping from 832 before, to 89 after treatment, whereas the cumulative relapse index (RI) dropped, during the same period, from 13.2 to 4.17 (P < 0.0001). No side effects were observed. It is concluded that patients with relapsing ocular herpes can benefit from treatment with HSV-specific TF.

[122]

Lawrence HS. Borkowsky W. **Transfer factor—current status and future prospects.** Biotherapy. 9(1-3):1-5, 1996.

We have detected new clues to the composition and function of "Transfer Factor" using the direct Leucocyte Migration Inhibition (LMI) test as an in vitro assay of Dialysates of Leucocyte Extracts (DLE). This approach has revealed two opposing antigen-specific activities to be present in the same > 3500 < 12,000 DA dialysis fraction - one activity is possessed of Inducer/Helper function (Inducer Factor). The opposing activity is possessed of Suppressor function (Suppressor Factor). When non-immune leucocyte populations are cultured with Inducer Factor they acquire the capacity to respond to specific antigen and inhibition of migration occurs. This conversion to reactivity is antigen-specific and dose-dependent. When immune leucocyte populations are cultured with Suppressor Factor their response to specific antigen is blocked and Inhibition of Migration is prevented.

[123]

Dwyer JM. **Transfer factor in the age of molecular biology: a review**. Biotherapy. 9(1-3):7-11, 1996.

Current data suggests that the transferring of immunologically specific information by transfer factor molecules requires interaction with a cell that has been genetically programmed to be antigen reactive but at the time of interaction is unprimed. Contact with transfer factor molecules would allow a naive recipient, on a first encounter with antigen, to make a secondary rather than a primary immunological response. Transfer factor molecules for each and every antigenic determinant are thus necessary. Transfer factors made from animals or humans are capable of transferring antigen specificity across a species barrier. Even primitive species have cells from which one can make transfer factors. The molecules are, therefore, well conserved and it is reasonable to suggest that they are important for normal immunological functioning. Proposed mechanisms of action must explain the fact that transfer factors obtained from the cells of high responder animals are capable of transferring delayed hypersensitivity to low responder animals while the reverse is not true. Transfer factor molecules are likely to interact with the variable regions of the alpha and/or beta chain of T cell receptors to change their avidity and affinity for antigen in a way that otherwise would only occur after an encounter with antigen.

[124]

Viza D. **AIDS and transfer factor: myths, certainties and realities**. Biotherapy. 9(1-3):17-26, 1996.

At the end of the 20th century, the triumph of biology is as indisputable as that of physics was at the end of the 19th century, and so is the might of the inductive thought. Virtually all diseases have been seemingly conquered and HIV, the cause of AIDS, has been fully described ten years after the onset of the epidemic. However, the triumph of biological science is far from being complete. The toll of several diseases, such as cancer, continues to rise and the pathogenesis of AIDS remains elusive. In the realm of inductive science, the dominant paradigm can seldom be challenged in a frontal attack, especially when it is apparently successful, and only what Kuhn calls "scientific revolutions" can overthrow it. Thus, it is hardly surprising that the concept of transfer factor is considered with contempt, and the existence of the moiety improbable: over forty years after the introduction of the concept, not only its molecular structure remains unknown, but also its putative mode of action contravenes dogmas of both immunology and molecular biology. And when facts challenge established dogmas, be in religion, philosophy or science, they must be suppressed. Thus, results of heterodox research become henceforth nisi-i.e., valid unless cause is shown for rescinding them, because they challenge the prevalent paradigm. However, when observations pertain to lethal disorders, their suppression in the name of dogmas may become criminal. Because of the failure of medical science to manage the AIDS pandemic, transfer factor, which has been successfully used for treating or preventing viral infections, may today overcome a priori prejudice and rejection more swiftly. In science, as in life, certainties always end up by dying, and Copernicus' vision by replacing that of Ptolemy.

[125]

Pizza G. Chiodo F. Colangeli V. Gritti F. Raise E. Fudenberg HH. De Vinci C. Viza D. **Preliminary observations using HIV-specific transfer factor in AIDS.** Biotherapy. 9(1-3):41-7, 1996.

Twenty five HIV-1-infected patients, at various stages (CDC II, III and IV) were treated orally with HIV-1-specific transfer factor (TF) for periods varying from 60 to 1870 days. All patients were receiving antiviral treatments in association with TF. The number of lymphocytes, CD4 and CD8 subsets were followed and showed no statistically significant variations. In 11/25 patients the number of lymphocytes increased, whilst in 11/25 decreased; similarly an increase of the CD4 lymphocytes was observed in 11/25 patients and of the CD8 lymphocytes in 15/25. Clinical improvement or a stabilized clinical condition was noticed in 20/25 patients, whilst a deterioration was seen in 5/25. In 12/14 anergic patients, daily TF administration restored delayed type hypersensitivity to recall antigens within 60 days. These preliminary observations suggest that oral HIV-specific TF administration, in association with antiviral drugs, is well tolerated and seems beneficial to AIDS patients, thus warranting further investigation.

[126]

Raise E. Guerra L. Viza D. Pizza G. De Vinci C. Schiattone ML. Rocaccio L. Cicognani M. Gritti F. **Preliminary results in HIV-1-infected patients treated with transfer factor (TF) and zidovudine (ZDV).** Biotherapy. 9(1-3):49-54, 1996.

The efficiency of HIV-1 specific transfer factor (TF) administration, combined with Zidovudine (ZDV), in asymptomatic persistent generalised lymphadenopaty, or AIDS related complex (ARC) patients was evaluated. Twenty patients were randomly assigned to receive only ZDV (1st group) or ZDV together with HIV-1-specific TF (2nd group). HIV-1-specific TF was administered orally at $2 \times 10(7)$ cell equivalent daily for 15 days, and thereafter once a week for up to 6 months. There were no significant differences between the two groups in clinical evolution, red blood cells, haemoglobin, lymphocytes, CD20 subset, transaminases, beta-2-microglobulin, p24 antigen. White blood cells, CD8 lymphocytes as well as IL-2 levels increased in the second group, while the CD4 subset increased in the first group. The combination treatment with ZDV and TF appeared to be safe and well tolerated. Furthermore, levels of serum cytokines were investigated in 10 patients (8 asymptomatic and 2 ARC) treated with ZDV, and compared with 5 patients of the 2nd group (3 asymptomatic and 2 ARC) treated with ZDV plus HIV-1-specific TF. Peripheral lymphocytes, CD4, CD8 subsets, IL-2, TNF alpha, IL-6, p24 antigen, IL-2 soluble lymphocyte receptors (sR), CD4sR, CD8sR and beta-2-microglobulin were evaluated at the baseline and at the 3rd month. The CD4 subset was not significantly different in the two groups, whilst IL-2 increased in the 2nd group receiving ZDV plus TF, suggesting an activation of the Th1 secretion pattern.

[127]

Fudenberg HH. **Dialysable lymphocyte extract (DLyE) in infantile onset autism: a pilot study.** Source Biotherapy. 9(1-3):143-7, 1996.

Abstract 40 infantile autistic patients were studied. They ranged from 6 years to 15 years of age at entry. 22 were cases of classical infantile autism; whereas 18 lacked one or more clinical defects associated with infantile autism ("pseudo-autism"). Of the 22 with classic autism, 21 responded to transfer factor (TF) treatment by gaining at least 2 points in symptoms severity score average (SSSA); and 10 became normal in that they were mainstreamed in school and clinical characteristics were fully normalized. Of the 18 remaining, 4 responded to TF, some to other therapies. After cessation of TF therapy, 5 in the autistic group and 3 of the pseudo-autistic group regressed, but they did not drop as low as baseline levels.

[128]

De Vinci, C. Pizza, G. Cuzzocrea, D. Menniti, D. Aiello, E. Maver, P. Corrado, G. Romagnoli, P. Dragoni, E. LoConte, G. Riolo, U. Masi, M. Severini, G. Fornarola, V. Viza, D. **Use of transfer factor for the treatment of recurrent non-bacterial female cystitis (NBRC): a preliminary report.** Biotherapy. 9(1-3):133-8, 1996.

Results of conventional treatment of female non-bacterial recurrent cystitis (NBRC) are discouraging. Most patients show an unexpected high incidence of vaginal candidiasis, while their cell mediated immunity to Herpes simplex viruses (HSV) and Candida antigens seems impaired, and it is known that the persistence of mucocutaneous chronic candidiasis is mainly due to a selective defect of CMI to Candida antigens. Twenty nine women suffering of NBRC, and in whom previous treatment with antibiotics and non-steroid anti-inflammatory drugs was unsuccessful, underwent oral transfer factor (TF) therapy. TF specific to Candida and/or to HSV was administered bi-weekly for the first 2 weeks, and then once a week for the following 6 months. No side effects were observed during treatment. The total observation period of our cohort was 24379 days with 353 episodes of cystitis recorded and a cumulative relapse index (RI) of 43. The observation period during and after treatment was 13920 days with 108 relapses and a cumulative RI of 23 (P < 0.0001). It, thus, seems that specific TF may be capable of controlling NBRC and alleviate the symptoms.

[130]

Liubchenko TA. Holeva OH. Kholodna LS. Smirnov VV. Vershyhora AIu. **The biological activity of the transfer factor induced by bacterial antigens** [Ukrainian] Mikrobiolohichnyi Zhurnal. 59(5):83-100, 1997.

Today's statement of transfer factor, an immunostimulator derived from leukocytes which enhances antiinfectious immunity, is observed in the review. Basic biological, physical and chemical characteristics of the transfer factor, its possible action mechanisms, and laboratory and clinical methods of use to cure infectious fungal (Candida, Coccidium), invasive (schistosomiasis, leishmaniasis, cryptosporidiosis), viral (varicella zoster, ophthalmic herpes, Herpes simplex types 1 and 2, H. zoster, H. simplex ceratitis, genital herpes, human herpes virus type 6, postherpetic neuritis, hepatitis B, AIDS), and bacterial infections (Mycobacterium leprae, M. tuberculosis, M. fortuitum, Salmonella cholerae suis, S. dublin, S. Virchov, Brucella abortus, Actinobacillus pleuropneumoniae, bacterial sepsis, Staphylococcus) are described.

[131]

Simko M. Mokran V. Nyulassy S. **Immunomodulatory therapy of epilepsy with transfer factor.** Bratislavske Lekarske Listy. 98(4):234-7, 1997.

Effect of immunotherapy with Transfer factor administered for a period of three months was studied in a group of ten epileptic patients, treated with carbamazepine or primidon previously and throughout the study. Out of eight patients, who finished the study we could notice significant reduction of epileptic discharges in eight patients. The results of this study prove that addition of immunomodulatory treatment to patients with intractable epilepsy could substantially improve the course of the disease in some patients.

[132]

Estrada-Parra S. Nagaya A. Serrano E. Rodriguez O. Santamaria V. Ondarza R. Chavez R. Correa B. Monges A. Cabezas R. Calva C. **Estrada-Garcia I. Comparative study of transfer factor and acyclovir in the treatment of herpes zoster.** International Journal of Immunopharmacology. 20(10):521-35, 1998.

Reactivation of varicella herpes virus (VHV), latent in individuals who have previously suffered varicella, gives rise to herpes zoster and in some cases leads to a sequela of post herpetic neuritis with severe pain which is refractory to analgesics. Many different antiviral agents have been tried without achieving satisfactory results. Of all the antiviral agents employed, acyclovir has been the most successful in reducing post herpetic pain. However acyclovir has not been as reliable as interferon alpha (IFN-alpha). We have previously looked into the use of transfer factor (TF) as a modulator of the immune system, specifically with respect to its effectiveness in the treatment of herpes zoster. In this work findings from a comparative clinical evaluation are presented. A double blind clinical trial of TF vs acyclovir was carried out in which 28 patients, presenting acute stage herpes zoster, were randomly assigned to either treatment group. Treatment was administered for seven days and the patients were subsequently submitted to daily clinical observation for an additional 14 days. An analogue visual scale was implemented in order to record pain and thereby served as the clinical parameter for scoring results. The group treated with TF was found to have a more favorable clinical course, P < or = 0.015. Laboratory tests to assess the immune profile of the patients were performed two days prior and 14 days after initial treatment. The results of these tests showed an increase in IFN-gamma levels, augmentation in the CD4+ cell population but not the percentage of T rosettes in the TF treated group. These parameters were however insignificantly modified in patients receiving acyclovir. Although TF treated patients showed an increase in CD4+ counts these cells remained below the levels for healthy individuals. The fact that IFN-gamma levels as well as the counts for CD4+ cells rose in the TF treated group and not in the acyclovir one is very significant and confirms the immunomodulating properties of TF.

[133]
Iushkova TA. Iushkov VV. **The immunomodulating activity of a transfer-factor preparation transflavin, specific to tick-borne encephalitis virus.** [Russian] Zhurnal Mikrobiologii, Epidemiologii i Immunobiologii. (2):83-5, 1998

Transflavin, a transfer-factor preparation specific to tick-borne encephalitis virus, was experimentally shown to possess immunomodulating action. The immunomodulating action of this preparation could be observed in a dose of 1 D (1 D being equivalent to 5 x 10(8) lymphocytes), which was manifested by an increase in the phagocytic activity of neutrophils and macrophages, a rise in the amount of T-lymphocytes, an increase in rosette formation, the number of antibody-forming cells, increased proliferation on T- and, to a lesser extent, B-cell mitogens, the restoration of the T-dependent expression of lymphocyte receptors, inhibited by trypsin. Transflavin in doses of 0, 1 and 10 D suppressed primary immune response. The probable mechanisms of the immunomodulating action of the Transflavin under study is discussed.

[134]

Cordero Miranda MA. Flores Sandoval G. Orea Solano M. Estrada Parra S. Serrano Miranda E. **Safety and efficacy of treatment for severe atopic dermatitis with cyclosporin A and transfer factor.** [Spanish]
Revista Alergia Mexico. 46(2):49-57, 1999.

The atopic dermatitis is a chronic skin disease that appears in patients with a personal or family history of allergic asthma and rhinitis. It is associated to the specific activation of a gene group. In most instances, the response to the conventional treatment is adequate. There are cases, though, know as refractory, where that is not the case. The study of two therapeutic alternatives, Transfer Factor (TF) and Cyclosporin A (CyA), was elaborated for this type of patients. MATERIAL AND METHODS: Patients with severe refractory AD were studied, being admitted to the Allergic Service to the ISSSTE Lic. Adolfo Lopez Mateos, ISSSTE, between September 1997 and june 1998. They were randomly divided in two groups. The first one was subjected to CyA, on a 4 mg/kg/day dosage, with monthly surveillance of kidney and hepatic functions and blood pressure twice a week. Group two was subjected to TF, as follows: one unit every third day for the first week, two units per week for the next three weeks and one monthly unit to complete six months. Initial and final clinical and immunologic testing was performed on both groups (eosinophils, total IgE, CD4 and CD8). RESULTS: Six patients included group A, and 12 patients in group B. Both groups showed a significant statistic reduction in the total eosinophils count, without an statistic difference between them. None showed changes in the total IgE. CyA reduced the CD4 levels, while the TF increased the levels of CD8 cells, both with a $p < 0.05$. Both groups showed clinical improvement satistically significant, but no differences with a $p > 0.05$ appeared between them. Tolerance to the treatments was adequate, and there was not need to suspend the treatment in any case. Only three patients showed hypertricosis and other one presented headaches, with CyA. CONCLUSION: Both treatments showed therapeutic benefits in the treatment of patients with severe refractory AD, with similar immunologic improvement. Both drugs present different action mechanisms, so their joint application could offer clinical benefit to the patient (synergetic action), cost reduction, and long term treatments with reduced adverse effects.

[135]

Kirkpatrick CH. **Transfer factors: identification of conserved sequences in transfer factor molecules**. Molecular Medicine. 6(4):332-41, 2000.

BACKGROUND: Transfer factors are small proteins that "transfer" the ability to express cell-mediated immunity from immune donors to non-immune recipients. We developed a process for purifying specific transfer factors to apparent homogeneity. This allowed us to separate individual transfer factors from mixtures containing several transfer factors and to demonstrate the antigen-specificity of transfer factors. Transfer factors have been shown to be an effective means for correction of deficient cellular immunity in patients with opportunistic infections, such as candidiasis or recurrent Herpes simplex and to provide prophylactic immunity against varicella-zoster in patients with acute leukemia. MATERIALS AND METHODS: Transfer factors of bovine and murine origin were purified by affinity chromatography and high performance liquid chromatography. Cyanogen bromide digests were sequenced. The properties of an apparently conserved sequence on expression of delayed-type hypersensitivity by transfer factor recipients were assessed. RESULTS: A novel amino acid sequence, LLYAQDL/VEDN, was identified in each of seven transfer factor preparations. These peptides would not transfer expression of delayed-type hypersensitivity to recipients, which indicates that they are not sufficient for expression of the specificity or immunological properties of native transfer factors. However, administration of the peptides to recipients of native transfer factors blocked expression of delayed-type hypersensitivity by the recipients. The peptides were not immunosuppressive. CONCLUSIONS: These findings suggest that the peptides may represent the portion of transfer factors that binds to the "target cells" for transfer factors. Identification of these cells will be helpful in defining the mechanisms of action of transfer factors.

[136]

Vacek A. Hofer M. Barnet K. Cech K. Pekarek J. Schneiderova H. **Positive effects of dialyzable leukocyte extract (DLE) on recovery of mouse haemopoiesis suppressed by ionizing radiation and on proliferation of haemopoietic progenitor cells in vitro.** International Journal of Immunopharmacology. 22(8):623-34, 2000.

Dialyzed leukocyte extract (DLE) (Immodin SEVAC, Czech Republic) was shown to enhance the recovery of the pools of hemopoietic stem cells (CFUs) and of granulocyte-macrophage hemopoietic progenitor cells (GM-CFC) in the bone marrow in vivo, as well as to increase the numbers of leukocytes and thrombocytes in the peripheral blood of mice exposed to a sublethal dose of gamma-rays, with an ensuing increase in the numbers of mice surviving the lethal radiation dose. In experiments performed in vitro, DLE or sera of mice administered with DLE were added to cultures of intact mouse bone marrow cells containing suboptimal concentrations of hemopoietic stimulatory cytokines, namely recombinant mouse interleukin-3 (rmIL-3) or recombinant mouse granulocyte-macrophage colony-stimulating factor (rmGM-CSF); under these experimental conditions, both DLE and sera of mice administered DLE were found to increase the counts of GM-CFC colonies in the cultures. It can be hypothesized on the basis of the findings obtained in vitro that the described co-stimulating activity (CoSA) of DLE may play a role also under in vivo conditions; the enhancement of the recovery of hemopoiesis suppressed by ionizing radiation may be due to a co-operation of the stimulatory effects of DLE with the action of cytokines endogenously produced in irradiated tissues.

[137]

Ojeda MO. Fernandez-Ortega C. Rosainz MJ. **Dialyzable leukocyte extract suppresses the activity of essential transcription factors for HIV-1 gene expression in unstimulated MT-4 cells.** Biochemical & Biophysical Research Communications. 273(3):1099-103, 2000 Jul 14.

The human immunodeficiency virus type 1 (HIV-1) contains regulatory regions in its long terminal repeat (LTR) implicated in the control of viral gene expression. We previously demonstrated that Dialyzable Leukocyte Extract (DLE), a preparation derived from immune leukocytes, is able to inhibit HIV-1 replication in MT-4 cell cultures. Here, we examined the effect of DLE on the activation of NF-kappaB and Sp1 transcription factors. NF-kappaB activity was completely suppressed after seven days of treatment with 2.5 U/mL of DLE, with a parallel large reduction in the amounts of Sp1 complexes. These findings correlate with the maximum inhibitory effect on HIV-1 replication described in a previous report. IkappaBalpha and NF-kappaB p65(RelA) gene expression are not regulated by DLE in MT-4 cells. Although up to day, the precise molecular mechanism of DLE biological activity in HIV-1 infection remains unclear, this report presents data that indicate a potential downregulatory effect of DLE on HIV-1 gene expression. Copyright 2000 Academic Press.

[138]

Sosa M. Flores G. Estrada S. Orea M. Gomez Vera J. **Comparative treatment between thalidomide and transfer factor in severe atopic dermatitis.** [Spanish] Revista Alergia Mexico. 48(2):56-64, 2001.

AIMS: The atopic dermatitis is an chronic inflammatory illness of the skin. It exists an interrelation complex of factors gene, environmental, and psychological that contribute to the development and severity of the illness. The immunol aberrations significant is the answer increased of IgE specific antibodies toward antigens common, the liberation is increased of immunol mediators by the basophils and mast cells, eosinophils peripheral and local, besides enlarges the biphasic activity Th1/Th2 with liberation of cytokines (IL-4, IL-5, IL-13), GM-C5F, and decrease of IFN-gamma by the cells Th1. Leung to report a knowledge upon the bases immunopathologies of it atopic dermatitis has immunopathologies clinical important for the diagnosis and processing. Alternatives multiples of processing by the same complexity of the illness exist. OBJECTIVE: To compare the security and the clinical efficacy of the thalidomide and the factor of transfer in the atopic dermatitis severe. MATERIAL AND METHOD: Were studied patient with diagnosis of atopic dermatitis severe in agreement with the criterions of Hanifin and Rajka that they entered to the service of Allergy and Immunology Clinical of the Hospital Regional Lic. Adolfo Lopez Mateos (public hospital). They were included 19 patient (women 12 and men 7, with age average 30 +/- 4 years). They were distributed in two groups. The first group of 5 patient administration thalidomide 200 mg/d during six months. The second group am administered the factor of transfer a total of 15 units by road oral during six months. Studies of laboratory for appraisal were requested immunology and metabolic pretreatment and pretreatment. RESULTS: In the group A dealt with thalidomide 5 patient and the group B dealt with FT, both presented a statistically significant decrease, as for the extension of the wounds (p < 0.01), and 1 am observed greater reduction in the intensity of the symptoms, the SCORAD total (p < 0.001 and p < 0.001 respectively) with statistical difference among them. None presented alterations immunologies and metabolic secondary to the use of the two drugs and not there was the need to suspend the processing. During the period of study, the patient were maintained controlled to the allergic rhinitis and the asthma. DISCUSSION: In the atopic dermatitis by its secondary clinical complexity to the multifactors etiologic, the alternatives of processing utilized in the present study are an option the security and efficacy, I am observed better clinical.

[139]

Franco-Molina MA. Mendoza-Gamboa E. Castillo-Leon L. Tamez-Guerra RS. Rodriguez-Padilla C. **Bovine dialyzable leukocyte extract protects against LPS-induced, murine endotoxic shock.** International Immunopharmacology. 4(13):1577-86, 2004.

The pathophysiology of endotoxic shock is characterized by the activation of multiple pro-inflammatory genes and their products which initiate the inflammatory process. Endotoxic shock is a serious condition with high mortality. Bovine dialyzable leukocyte extract (bDLE) is a dialyzate of a heterogeneous mixture of low molecular weight substances released from disintegrated leukocytes of the blood or lymphoid tissue obtained from homogenized bovine spleen. bDLE is clinically effective for a broad spectrum of diseases. To determine whether bDLE improves survival and modulates the expression of pro-inflammatory cytokine genes in LPS-induced, murine endotoxic shock, Balb/C mice were treated with bDLE (1 U) after pretreatment with LPS (17 mg/kg). The bDLE improved survival (90%), suppressed IL-10 and IL-6, and decreased IL-1beta, TNF-alpha, and IL-12p40 mRNA expression; and decreased the production of IL-10 ($P<0.01$), TNF-alpha ($P<0.01$), and IL-6 ($P<0.01$) in LPS-induced, murine endotoxic shock. Our results demonstrate that bDLE leads to improved survival in LPS-induced endotoxic shock in mice, modulating the pro-inflammatory cytokine gene expression, suggesting that bDLE is an effective therapeutic agent for inflammatory illnesses associated with an unbalanced expression of proinflammatory cytokine genes such as in endotoxic shock, rheumatic arthritis and other diseases.

[140]

Fabre RA. Perez TM. Aguilar LD. Rangel MJ. Estrada-Garcia I. Hernandez-Pando R. Estrada Parra S. **Transfer factors as immunotherapy and supplement of chemotherapy in experimental pulmonary tuberculosis.** Clinical & Experimental Immunology. 136(2):215-23, 2004.

Problems of logistics, compliance and drug resistance point to an urgent need for immunotherapeutic strategies capable of shortening the current six month antibiotic regimens used to treat tuberculosis. One potential immunotherapeutic agent is transfer factors. Transfer factors (TF) are low molecular weight dialysable products from immune cells which transmit the ability to express delayed-type hypersensitivity (DTH) and cell mediated immunity from sensitized donors to nonimmune recipients. In this study we determined the efficiency of TF as immunotherapy to treat experimental tuberculosis. When BALB/c mice are infected via the trachea with Mycobacterium tuberculosis H37Rv there is an initial phase of partial resistance dominated by Th-1 type cytokines plus tumour necrosis factor-alpha (TNFalpha) and the inducible isoform of nitric oxide synthase (iNOS), followed by a phase of progressive disease characterized by increasing expression of IL-4, diminished expression of TNFalpha and iNOS, and low DTH. Animals in this late progressive phase of the disease (day 60) were treated with different doses of TF (one injection per week) obtained from spleen cells when the peak of immune protection in this animal model is reached (day 21), or with different doses of TF from peripheral leucocytes of PPD + healthy subjects. We show here that the treatment with murine or human TF restored the expression of Th-1 cytokines, TNFalpha and iNOS provoking inhibition of bacterial proliferation and significant increase of DTH and survival. This beneficial effect was dose dependent. Interestingly, murine TF in combination with conventional chemotherapy had a synergistic effect producing significant faster elimination of lung bacteria loads than chemotherapy alone.

[141]

Orozco TT. Solano MO. Sandoval GF. Vera JG. Parra SE. **Inflammatory mediators in patients with atopic dermatitis after treatment with transfer factor.** [Spanish] Revista Alergia Mexico. 51(4):151-4, 2004.

BACKGROUND: Atopic dermatitis is a skin inflammatory disease, which is associated to high levels of IgE, eosinophiles and change of T lymphocytes. OBJECTIVE: To determine if the treatment with transfer factor for moderate atopic dermatitis decreases the number of inflammatory cells in the peripheral blood. MATERIAL AND METHODS: We selected twenty patients with diagnosis of moderate atopic dermatitis. The age range of the patients was between 5 and 45 years old. Patients were assigned to one of three groups: group A included patients with atopic dermatitis treated with transfer factor: one unit a day for five days, two units a week, one unit a week, one unit every fifteen days and one unit a month. Group B included ten patients with atopic dermatitis who received conventional treatment (hydrox-yzine 10 mg/24 h) and the group C was conformed by healthy controls. All patients were submitted to basal and final determination of IgE, peripheral blood eosinophils, and underpopulation of lymphocytes by flow cytometry. Study period was of ten weeks. RESULTS: Levels of IgE were reduced respect to the basal value. In the patients of group A there was an increase in neutrophils and leukocytes after treatment; however, it was not significant ($p = 0.46$). Eosinophils were significantly reduced ($p = 0.01$). After comparing group A to group C the p value was of 0.035. CONCLUSION: In patients with atopic dermatitis, after 10 weeks of treatment with transfer factor, the level of IgE and peripheral eosinophils was reduced.

[142]

Fernandez-Ortega C. Dubed M. Ramos Y. Navea L. Alvarez G. Lobaina L. Lopez L. Casillas D. Rodriguez L. **Non-induced leukocyte extract reduces HIV replication and TNF secretion.** Biochemical & Biophysical Research Communications. 325(3):1075-81, 2004.

According to UNAIDS, the global HIV/AIDS epidemic increased to 40 million the number of people living with the virus around the world. Dialyzable leukocyte extract obtained by our group is a low molecular weight dialyzable material from peripheral human leukocytes previously in vitro induced with Sendai virus (DLE-ind), and more recently, from non-induced leukocytes (DLE n/i). Previous results have shown the ability of DLE-ind to inhibit HIV in vitro replication in MT4 cell; to reduce TNFalpha secretion, and to delay in vivo progression to AIDS in early stage of HIV infection. In this work we present evidences that DLE n/i also inhibits HIV in vitro replication and reduces TNFalpha secretion in human whole blood like DLE obtained from induced leukocytes. Taking together these results show that both properties of DLE, HIV in vitro inhibition and TNF production modulation, are not dependent on in vitro Sendai virus induction of leukocytes.

[143]

Flores Sandoval G. Gomez Vera J. Orea Solano M. Lopez Tiro J. Serrano E. Rodriguez A. Rodriguez A. Estrada Parra S. Jimenez Saab N. **Transfer factor as specific immunomodulator in the treatment of moderate-severe atopic dermatitis.** [Spanish] Revista Alergia Mexico. 52(6):215-20, 2005.

BACKGROUND: Atopic dermatitis is a skin inflammatory disease which has been associated to high levels of IgE, eosinophiles and change of T lymphocytes. The transfer factor is an immunomodulator active substance and decreases the number of inflammatory cells and the severity of the symptoms of atopic dermatitis. OBJECTIVE: To determine the efficacy of the transfer factor as treatment of moderate and severe atopic dermatitis. MATERIAL AND METHODS: Articles related to treatment with transfer factor in the atopic dermatitis were looked up in Medline and EMBASE, and the ones referring to controlled studies in patients with moderate and severe atopic dermatitis in accord to SCORAD. RESULTS: We found seven articles with 121 patients and 88 controls demonstrating significant decrease in the symptoms of the SCORAD index, decreased IgE, and eosinophils in patients treated with transfer factor. CONCLUSIONS: The transfer factor is a choice treatment for moderate and severe atopic dermatitis.

[144]

Franco-Molina MA. Mendoza-Gamboa E. Castillo-Leon L. Tamez-Guerra RS. Rodriguez-Padilla C. **Bovine dialyzable leukocyte extract modulates the nitric oxide and pro-inflammatory cytokine production in lipopoly-saccharide-stimulated murine peritoneal macrophages in vitro.** Journal of Medicinal Food. 8(1):20-6, 2005.

Lipopolysaccharides (LPS) released from Gram-negative bacteria after infection initiate an exagerated response that leads to a cascade of pathophysiological events termed sepsis. Monocytes or macrophages produce many of the mediators found in septic patients. Targeting of these mediators, especially tumor necrosis factor (TNF)-alpha and nitric oxide (NO), has been pursued as a mean of reducing mortality in sepsis. Bovine dialyzable leukocyte extract (bDLE) is a dialysate of a heterogeneous mixture of low-molecular-weight substances released from disintegrated leukocytes of the blood or tissue lymphoid. In this study, to determine whether bDLE modulates NO and pro-inflammatory cytokine production, murine peritoneal macrophages were treated with bDLE (0.05 or 0.5 U/mL) before LPS (20 mg/mL) stimulation, and also LPS-stimulated murine peritoneal macrophages were treated with bDLE (0.05 or 0.5 U/mL) at 0, 4, 8, 12, and 24 hours. The bDLE significantly decreased NO production, and also decreased TNF-alpha and interleukin (IL)-6 but increased IL-10 production in LPS-stimulated murine peritoneal macrophages. Our results demonstrate that bDLE plays an important role in modulating TNF-alpha, IL-6, and NO production through IL-10, and this may offer therapeutic potential in clinical endotoxic shock.

[145]

Pineda B. Estrada-Parra S. Pedraza-Medina B. Rodriguez-Ropon A. Perez R. Arrieta O. **Interstitial transfer factor as adjuvant immunotherapy for experimental glioma.** Journal of Experimental & Clinical Cancer Research. 24(4):575-83, 2005.

Glioblastoma multiform (GBM) is the most common tumour of the central nervous system in humans. Unfortunately its prognosis is poor and because of the lack of efficacious therapies, immunotherapy is a potential treatment. Transfer factors (TF) are low molecular weight dialysable products extracted from immune cells which transmit the ability to express delayed-type hypersensitivity and cell mediated immunity from sensitized donors to nonimmnune recipients. In this study, we determined the efficacy of TF as immunotherapy to treat experimental glioblastoma. We used TF obtained from immunized swine. We evaluated different doses of intratumoral TF (product of 4x10(6), 8x10(5) and 1.6x10(5) cells). The best dose (product of 4x10(6) cells) of TF was also combined with carmustine for experimental therapy in rats with C6 malignant glioma. Modifications in peripheral blood T lymphocyte counts (CD2+, CD4+, CD8+ and NK) were evaluated by flow cytometry. Cytokine expression in the tumour was assessed by RT-PCR and apoptosis was evaluated using the sub G0 method. Intratumoral TF reduced significantly the tumour size, and increased CD2+, CD4+, CD8+ and NK cell counts, it also increased the percentage of apoptotic tumour cells and the percentage of tumour tissue expressing Th1 cytokines. We observed an additive antitumoral effect when TF was combined with chemotherapy.

[146]

Ojeda MO. van't Veer C. Fernandez Ortega CB. Arana Rosainz Mde J. Buurman WA. **Dialyzable leukocyte extract differentially regulates the production of TNFalpha, IL-6, and IL-8 in bacterial component-**

activated leukocytes and endothelial cells. Inflammation Research. 54(2):74-81, 2005.

OBJECTIVE: To investigate i) whether the Dialyzable Leukocyte Extract (DLE) modulates the production of proinflammatory cytokines in leukocytes activated by the bacterial cell wall components lipopolysaccharide (LPS), lipoteichoic acid (LTA), and peptidoglycan (PGN); ii) the effect of DLE on LPS-stimulated endothelial cells; and iii) whether the regulatory effect of DLE on inflammatory mediators is related to the modulation of Toll-like receptors (TLRs), NF-kappaB and cAMP signaling pathways. METHODS: Leukocytes were stimulated with LPS, LTA, and PGN in the presence of DLE. Endothelial cells were stimulated with LPS and treated with DLE. The levels of Tumor Necrosis Factor-alpha (TNFalpha), Interleukin-6 (IL-6), and IL-8 in culture supernatants were evaluated by ELISA. The expression of Toll-like receptor 2 (TLR2) and 4 (TLR4), NF-kappaB activity and cAMP levels were evaluated by flow cytometry, EMSA, and EIA, respectively. RESULTS: The addition of DLE to leukocytes stimulated with cell wall constituents suppressed the production of TNFalpha. However, DLE induced IL-8 release in monocytes and enhanced IL-6 and IL-8 production by activated monocytes and endothelial cells. Also, DLE induced TLR2 and TLR4 expression, and increased cAMP levels, whereas NF-kappaB activity was inhibited. CONCLUSIONS: The present data indicate the differential regulation by DLE of the production of TNFalpha, IL-6, and IL-8 cytokines, associated with effects on TLR2 and TLR4 expression and NF-kappaB and cAMP activities. We suggest a putative mechanism for the biological effects of DLE in activated leukocytes and endothelial cells.

[147]

Armides Franco-Molina M. Mendoza-Gamboa E. Castillo-Tello P. Tamez-Guerra RS. Villarreal-Trevino L. Tijerina-Menchaca R. Castillo-Leon L. Zapata-Benavides P. Rodriguez-Padilla C. **In vitro antibacterial activity of bovine dialyzable leukocyte extract.** Immunopharmacology & Immunotoxicology. 28(3):471-83, 2006.

The rapidly developing resistance of many infectious pathogenic organisms to modern drugs has spurred scientists to search for new sources of antibacterial compounds. One potential candidate, bDLE (dialysis at 10 to 12 kDa cut-off) and its fractions ("S" and "L" by 3.5 kDa cut-off and I, II, III, and IV by molecular exclusion chromatography), was evaluated for antibacterial activity against pathogenic bacterial strains (Staphylococcus aureus, Streptococcus pyogenes, Lysteria monocytogenes, Escherichia coli, Pseudomonas aeruginosa, and Salmonella typhi) using standard antimicrobial assays. A minimum inhibitory concentration (MIC) of bDLE and its fractions was determined by agar and broth dilutions methods. Only bDLE and its "S" fraction had an effect upon all bacteria evaluated (MIC ranging from 0.29 to 0.62 U/ml), and the bactericidal and bacteriostatic effects (evaluated by MTT assay) were bacterial species-dependent. These results showed a remarkable in vitro antibacterial property of bDLE against several pathogenic bacteria.

[148]

Xu YP. Zou WM. Zhan XJ. Yang SH. Xie DZ. Peng SL. **Preparation and determination of immunological activities of anti-HBV egg yolk extraction.** Cellular & Molecular Immunology. 3(1):67-71, 2006.

To prepare an effective immune preparation to treat hepatitis B, hens were immunized with hepatitis B vaccines, and then anti-HBV egg yolk extraction (anti-HBV EYE) was refined from egg yolk by a dialyzable method. Its chemical characteristics were identified by ultraviolet spectrum, HPLC, Lowry analysis and pharmacopocia-raleted methods. The specific immunological activity was examined by leukocyte adherence inhibition (LAI) in vitro and delayed type hypersensitivity (DTH) in vivo. Anti-HBV EYE was a small dialyzable substance with molecular weight less than 12 kD containing 18 kinds of amino acids. The preparation could obviously inhibit LAI and DTH which was similar to hepatitis B virus-specific transfer factor of pig spleen. However, there were no similar effects observed in the nonspecific transfer factor (NTF) group, control egg yolk extraction (CEYE) group and hepatitis A virus (HAV) group. The results suggested that anti-HBV EYE contained hepatitis B virus-specific transfer factor (STF) and had the antigen-specific cell immune activity similar to PSHBV-TF. The STF obtained from egg yolk of the hens immunized with specific antigen, might be a potential candidate for immunoregulation in hepatitis B prevention and treatment.

[149]

Franco-Molina MA. Mendoza-Gamboa E. Miranda-Hernandez D. Zapata-Benavides P. Castillo-Leon L. Isaza-Brando C. Tamez-Guerra RS. Rodriguez-Padilla C. **In vitro effects of bovine dialyzable leukocyte extract (bDLE) in cancer cells.** Cytotherapy. 8(4):408-14, 2006.

BACKGROUND: Bovine dialyzable leukocyte extract (bDLE) is a dialyzate of a heterogeneous mixture of low molecular weight substances released from disintegrated blood leukocytes or lymphoid tissue obtained from homogenized bovine spleen. The purpose of this study was to determine if bDLE had cytotoxic effects and modulated apoptosis gene expression in breast cancer cells. METHODS: The MCF-7, BT-474, MDA-MB-453, A-427, Calu-1, U937 and L5178Y cancer cell lines and PBMC human cells were treated with bDLE (0-0.66 U/mL) for 72 h. The bDLE effect on cell growth proliferation was evaluated by MTT assay, and the MCF-7 was evaluated by ethidium bromide-acridine orange staining; total DNA was evaluated for

DNA fragmentation, and total RNA was isolated for p53, bag-1, c-myc, bim, bax, bcl-2 and bad mRNA expression. RESULTS: The bDLE had dose-dependent cytotoxic effects and demonstrated an IC50 at a dosage of 0.06 U/mL (P<0.05). The bDLE did not affect the viability of normal human PBMC. The bDLE induced DNA fragmentation at doses of 0.06 and 0.13 U/mL in MCF-7 breast cancer cells. The bDLE induced cytotoxic effects and suppressed the p53, bag-1, c-myc, bax, bcl-2, and bad mRNA expression that influences apoptosis in MCF-7 breast cancer cells. Bim mRNA expression was not detected. DISCUSSION: This may open up interesting prospects for the treatment of human breast cancer.

[150]

Abubakar, I. Aliyu, S H. Arumugam, C. Hunter, P R. Usman, N K. **Prevention and treatment of cryptosporidiosis in immunocompromised patients.** Cochrane Database of Systematic Reviews. (1):CD004932, 2007.

BACKGROUND: Cryptosporidiosis is a disease that causes diarrhoea lasting about one to two weeks, sometimes extending up to 2.5 months among the immunocompetent and becoming a more severe life-threatening illness among immunocompromised individuals. Cryptosporidium is a common cause of gastroenteritis. Cryptosporidiosis is common in HIV-infected individuals. OBJECTIVES: The objective of the review was to assess the efficacy of interventions for the treatment and prevention of cryptosporidiosis among immunocompromised individuals. SEARCH STRATEGY: We searched the following databases for randomised controlled trials up to August 2005: Cochrane Central Register of Controlled Trials (CENTRAL), MEDLINE, AIDSLINE, AIDSearch, EMBASE, CINAHL, Current Contents, Geobase, and the Environmental Sciences and Pollution Management. SELECTION CRITERIA: Randomised controlled trials that compared the use of any intervention to treat or prevent cryptosporidiosis in immunocompromised persons were included. The outcome measures for treatment studies included symptomatic diarrhoea and oocyst clearance. DATA COLLECTION AND ANALYSIS: Two reviewers independently assessed the trials for quality of randomisation, blinding, withdrawals, and adequacy of allocation concealment. The relative risk for each intervention was calculated using a random effects model. MAIN RESULTS: Seven trials involving 169 participants were included. There were 130 adults with AIDS enrolled in five studies. Evidence of significant heterogeneity was present. There was no evidence for a reduction in the duration or frequency of diarrhoea by nitazoxanide (RR 0.83 (95% CI 0.36-1.94)) and paramomycin (RR 0.74 (95% CI 0.42-1.31)) compared with placebo. Nitazoxanide led to a significant evidence of oocyst clearance compared with placebo among all children with a relative risk of 0.52 (95% CI 0.30-0.91). The effect was not significant for

HIV-seropositive participants (RR 0.71 (95% CI 0.36-1.37)). HIV-seronegative participants on nitazoxanide had a significantly higher relative risk of achieving parasitological clearance of 0.26 (95% CI 0.09-0.80) based on a single study. The single study comparing spiramycin with placebo found no significant difference in reduction of the duration of hospitalisation (mean difference -0.40 days (95% CI -6.62-5.82)) or in mortality between the two arms of the trial (RR 0.43 (95% CI 0.04-4.35)). One study assessed the role of bovine dialyzable leukocyte extract, reporting a relative risk for decreased stool frequency of 0.19 (95% CI 0.03-1.19), while another compared bovine hyperimmune colostrum with placebo and found no evidence for improvement of stool volume (RR 3.00 (95% CI 0.61-14.86)) or in oocyst concentration per ml of stool (RR 0.27 (95% CI 0.02-3.74)). No studies were found that assessed prevention. AUTHORS' CONCLUSIONS: This review confirms the absence of evidence for effective agents in the management of cryptosporidiosis. The results indicate that nitazoxanide reduces the load of parasites and may be useful in immunocompetent individuals. Due to the seriousness of the potential outcomes of cryptosporidiosis, the use of nitazoxanide should be considered in immunocompromised patients. The absence of effective therapy highlights the need to ensure that infection is avoided. Unfortunately, evidence for the effectiveness and cost-effectiveness of preventive intervene tions is also lacking.

[151]

Melenevs'ka NV, Miroshnychenko MC, Filippov IB, Kholodna LS, Shuba MF. **Transfer factor of immune reactivity to diphtheria-tetanus anatoxin modulates the action of neurotransmitters in the intestinal smooth muscle** [Article in Ukrainian] Fiziol Zh. 53(1):24-32, 2007

Transfer factor (TF) of immune reactivity ($10(-5)$ - $10(-3)$ mg/ml) to diphtheria-tetanus anatoxin modulates slow waves and spontaneous contractile activity of non-atropinized smooth muscle stripes (SMS) of guinea-pig taenia coli. TF ($10(-4)$ mg/ml) transforms slow waves into stable depolarization and tonic contraction. After SMS atropinization, the substance acts in the same way. In the presence of methylene blue ($10(-5)$ M), a guanylatecyclase blocker, FT induces transitory increase of SMS muscle tone, which is followed by their stable relaxation. ATP and UTP, purinoceptors agonists, evoke substantial hyperpolarization of smooth muscle cells membrane and their relaxation. FT enhances post-inhibitory excitation in SMS. In the presence of acetylcholine ($10(-5)$ M) FT ($10(-4)$ mg/ml) transforms the inhibitory ATP action on tonic contraction into excitative. This substance ($10(-5)$, $10(-4)$ mg/ml) enhances $Ca2+$ mobilization from ryanodine-sensitive calcium store, inhibits the release of these cations from IP3-sensitive calcium store of sarcoplasmic reticulum. TF demolishes the inhibitory actions of sodium nitroprusside (nitric oxide donor), and noradrenaline in taenia coli smooth muscles.

[152]

Franco-Molina MA, Mendoza-Gamboa E, Zapata-Benavides P, Vera-García ME, Castillo-Tello P, García de la Fuente A, Mendoza RD, Garza RG, Támez-Guerra RS, Rodríguez-Padilla C. **IMMUNEPOTENT CRP (bovine dialyzable leukocyte extract) adjuvant immunotherapy: a phase I study in non-small cell lung cancer patients.** Cytotherapy. 10(5):490-6, 2008

BACKGROUND: IMMUNEPOTENT CRP is a mixture of low molecular weight substances, some of which have been shown to be capable of modifying the immune response. We evaluated the response and adjuvant effect of IMMUNEPOTENT CRP on non-small cell lung cancer (NSCLC) patients in a phase I clinical trial. METHODS: Twenty-four NSCLC patients were included in the study and divided into two groups. Group 1 received a conventional treatment of 5400 cGy external radiotherapy in 28 fractions and chemotherapy consisting of intravenous cisplatin (40 mg/m(2)) delivered weekly for 6 weeks. Group 2 received the conventional treatment plus IMMUNEPOTENT CRP (5 U) administered daily. We performed clinical evaluation by CT scan and radiography analysis, and determined the quality of life of the patients with the Karnofsky performance scale. A complete blood count (red and white blood cell tests), including flow cytometry analysis, blood work (alkaline phosphatase test) and a delayed-type hypersensitivity (DTH) skin test for PPD, Varidase and Candida were performed. RESULTS: The administration of IMMUNEPOTENT CRP induced immunomodulatory activity (increasing the total leukocytes and T-lymphocyte subpopulations CD4(+), CD8(+), CD16(+) and CD56(+), and maintaining DHT) and increased the quality of the patients' lives, suggesting immunologic protection against chemotherapeutic side-effects in NSCLC patients. DISCUSSION: Our results suggest the possibility of using IMMUNEPOTENT CRP alongside radiation and chemotherapy for maintaining the immune system and increasing the quality of life of the patients.

[153]

Berrón-Pérez R, Chávez-Sánchez R, Estrada-García I, Espinosa-Padilla S, Cortez-Gómez R, Serrano-Miranda E, Ondarza-Aguilera R, Pérez-Tapia M, Pineda Olvera B, Jiménez-Martínez Mdel C, Portugués A, Rodríguez A, Cano L, Pacheco PU, Barrientos J, Chacón R, Serafín J, Mendez P, Monges A, Cervantes E, Estrada-Parra S. **Indications, usage, and dosage of the transfer factor.** Rev Alerg Mex. 54(4):134-9, 2007.

The transfer factor (TF) was described in 1955 by S. Lawrence. In 1992 Kirkpatrick characterized the specific TF at molecular level. The TF is constituted by a group of numerous molecules, of low molecular weight, from 1.0 to 6.0 kDa. The 5 kDa fraction corresponds to the TF specific to antigens. There are a number of publications about the clinical indications of the TF for diverse diseases, in particular those where the cellular immune response is compromised or in those where there is a deficient regulation of the immune response. In this article we present our clinical and basic experiences, especially regarding the indications, usage and dosage of the TF. Our group demonstrated that the TF increases the expression of IFN-gamma and RANTES, while decreases the expression of osteopontine. Using animal models we have worked with M. tuberculosis, and with a model of glioma with good therapeutic results. In the clinical setting we have worked with herpes zoster, herpes simplex type I, herpetic keratitis, atopic dermatitis, osteosarcoma, tuberculosis, asthma, post-herpetic neuritis, anergic coccidioidomycosis, leishmaniasis, toxoplasmosis, mucocutaneous candidiasis, pediatric infections produced by diverse pathogen germs, sinusitis, pharyngitis, and otits media. All of these diseases were studied through protocols which main goals were to study the therapeutic effects of the TF, and to establish in a systematic way diverse dosage schema and time for treatment to guide the prescription of the TF.

[154]

White A. **Why vaccines are not the answer - the failure of V520 and the importance of cell-mediated immunity in the fight against HIV**. Med Hypotheses. 71(6):909-13, 2008

The recent failure of Merck's HIV vaccine, V520, left the future of HIV vaccine research in question. The current article offers a possible explanation for the failure of V520 and explores a potential alternative to the vaccine approach. Vaccines prior to V520 were designed to evoke strong antibody-mediated immune responses to HIV; that is, the generation of antibodies to attach to and disable the HIV virus before it infiltrates host cells. V520 represents a misguided, though well-intentioned, effort to evoke a cell-mediated immune response to HIV; that is, immune activity aimed at identifying proteins associated with HIV after it infiltrates host cells. In the body, these two immune responses, antibody-mediated (for extracellular infections) and cell-mediated (primarily for intracellular infections), operate in a teeter-totter fashion. When one is activated the other is suppressed. Because HIV quickly infects host cells near entrances to the body, it requires a strong cell-mediated response to defeat, not an antibody-mediated response. The driving hypothesis of this article is that the antibody-mediated immune response triggered by V520 suppressed the ability of the body to mount the cell-mediated immune response necessary to protect against HIV and created a window of opportunity for HIV infection, particularly in subjects previously exposed to the adenovirus vector used in the vaccine. While the immune system uses antibodies to identify extracellular pathogens, it uses transfer factors to label infected host cells. Hundred of papers indicate that pathogen-specific transfer factors can be used to stimulate cell-mediated immunity against a wide variety of viruses. The available research, reviewed in this manuscript, suggests that HIV-specific transfer factors could prove extremely useful, far more useful than vaccines, in preventing and treating HIV infections.

[155]

Wang SJ, Jiao CY, Sun XD. **Clinical observation of effect of jiawei yupingfeng mixture for prevention and treatment of 100 children with repeated respiratory tract infection** [Article in Chinese]. Zhongguo Zhong Xi Yi Jie He Za Zhi. 2009;29(8):742-5.

OBJECTIVE: To investigate the effect of Jiawei Yupingfeng Mixture (YPF) on repeated respiratory tract infection (RRTI) and its impacts on T-cell subsets, immunoglobulin and erythrocyte immune. METHODS: Two hundred children with RRTI were assigned equally to two groups, the test group treated with YPF and the control group treated by transfer factor. The clinical efficacy, and the changes of T-cell subsets, immunoglobulin and erythrocyte immune before and after treatment were observed in 31 patients randomly selected from each group. RESULTS: After treatment, the frequency of attacking was reduced and the course of attacking was shortened significantly in the test group as compared with before treatment and also with the control group (P < 0.01); IgG and IgA levels were improved in both groups, but the improvement was more significant in the test group (P<0.01, P<0.05); T-cell subsets indices, including CD3(+), CD4(+), CD8(+) and CD4(+)/CD8(+) ratio, all improved in the test group significantly (P <0.01), while in the control group, significant improvement only showed in rising of CD3(+) and CD4(+) (P <0.05, P <0.01), comparison between groups showed significant difference in terms of CD3(+), CD4(+) and CD8(+); in the control group, levels of C3b, RFER and RFIR were changed significantly (P<0.05, P<0.01), but the improvement of ICR was insignificant, while in the test group, the above indices were significant improved as compared with after treatment of the control group (P <0.01). CONCLUSION: YPF plays a preventive and therapeatic role in children with RRTI by way of regulating the cellular and humoral immune.

[156]

Espinosa Padilla SE, Orozco S, Plaza A, Estrada Parra S, Estrada García I, Rosales González MG, Villaverde Rosa R, Espinosa Rosales FJ. **Effect of transfer factor on treatment with glucocorticoids in a group of pediatric**

patients with persistent moderate allergic asthma [Article in Spanish]. Rev Alerg Mex. 2009;56(3):67-71.

BACKGROUND: Inhaled glucocorticoids are the most effective and potent drugs used to control the inflammatory bronchial reaction in patients with asthma. There are several research projects evaluating the use of immune modulators in the treatment of the asthma related inflammatory process. OBJECTIVE: To evaluate the effect of transfer factor in the treatment of pediatric patients with moderate persistent allergic asthma in terms of inhaled glucocorticoid dosing and time of using. PATIENTS AND METHODS: Randomized, double blind, placebo controlled pilot clinical trial in a cohort of pediatric patients (6-17 years old) with moderate persistent allergic asthma. Two groups were formed. Group one received transfer factor and group two was given placebo. Both groups received conventional therapy with inhaled budesonide and formoterol. Daily respiratory symptoms (cough during day, or at night, and wheezing episodes) were recorded in a personal diary. Spirometric evaluations were performed before enrolling patients, and at 1, 3 and 6 months after. RESULTS: Eleven patients were enrolled in each group. Patients in the transfer factor group showed a statistical significant reduction in the inhaled glucocorticoid doping since month 3, and this difference was maintained until the end of study. Patients on TF group showed also a non statistical significant improvement in spirometrical findings and also showed a better asthma control. CONCLUSIONS: Transfer factor helps to reduce inhaled glucocorticoids dose in patients with allergic rhinitis; however, studies with a larger number of patients should be done in order to obtain better results.

[157]

Dvoroznáková E, Porubcová J, Sevcíková Z. **Immune response of mice with alveolar echinococcosis to therapy with transfer factor, alone and in combination with albendazole.** Parasitol Res. 2009;105(4):1067-76.

The effect of dialysable leucocyte extract (transfer factor TF) on immune response of mice infected with Echinococcus multilocularis and treated with albendazole (ABZ) was observed. TF administration increased the parasite-suppressed proliferative response of T and B lymphocytes of infected mice from weeks 8 to 12 or 14 post infection (p.i.), respectively, with the most stimulative effect after TF+ABZ therapy. The CD4 T cell presence in the spleen of infected mice with TF or TF+ABZ therapy was increased from weeks 6 to 12 or 14 p.i., respectively. The production of IFN-gamma (Th1 cytokine) after TF or TF+ABZ therapy was significantly higher from weeks 6 to 12 p.i., and during this time, the significantly inhibited IL-5 synthesis (Th2 cytokine) was detected, particularly after TF+ABZ therapy. The superoxide anion (O2-) production in peritoneal macrophages of infected mice treated with TF or TF+ABZ was stimulated from weeks 8 to 18 p.i. The immunomodulative effect of TF reduced the growth of larval cysts till week 14 p.i. with a comparable intensity to the anthelmintic drug ABZ. Combined therapy TF+ABZ resulted in the greatest parasite restriction and reduced the cyst development till the end of the experiment.

[158]*

Szaniszlo P, German P, Hajas G, Saenz DN, Kruzel M, Boldogh I. **New insights into clinical trial for Colostrinin in Alzheimer's disease.** J Nutr Health Aging. 2009;13(3):235-41.

BACKGROUND: The pathomechanism of Alzheimer's disease (AD) is multifactorial although the most popular hypotheses are centered on the effects of the misfolded, aggregated protein, amyloid beta (Abeta) and on Tau hyperphosphorylation. OBJECTIVES: Double blinded clinical trials were planned to demonstrate the effect of Colostrinin (CLN) on instrumental daily activities of AD patients. The potential molecular mechanisms by which CLN mediates its effects were investigated by gene expression profiling. METHODS: RNAs isolated from CLN-treated cells were analyzed by high-density oligonucleotide arrays. Network and pathway analyses were performed using the Ingenuity Pathway Analysis software. RESULTS: The Full Sample Analysis at week 15 showed a stabilizing effect of CLN on cognitive function in ADAS-cog (p = 0.02) and on daily function in IADL (p = 0.02). The overall patient response was also in favor of CLN (p = 0.03). Patients graded as mild on entry also showed a superior response of ADAS-cog compared to more advanced cases (p = 0.01). Data derived from microarray network analysis show that CLN elicits highly complex and multiphasic changes in the cells' transcriptome. Importantly, transcriptomal analysis showed that CLN alters gene expression of molecular networks implicated in Abeta precursor protein synthesis, Tau phosphorylation and increased levels of enzymes that proteolytically eliminate Abeta. In addition, CLN enhanced the defense against oxidative stress and decreased expression of inflammatory chemokines and cytokines, thereby attenuating inflammatory processes that precede Alzheimer's and other neurological diseases. CONCLUSION: Together these data suggest that CLN has promising potential for clinical use in prevention and therapy of Alzheimer's and other age-associated central nervous system diseases.

[159]*

Douraghi-Zadeh D, Matharu B, Razvi A, Austen B. **The protective effects of the nutraceutical, colostrinin, against Alzheimer's disease, is mediated via prevention of apoptosis in human neurones induced by aggregated beta-amyloid.** J Nutr Health Aging. 2009;13(6):522-7.

OBJECTIVE: It has previously been demonstrated that oral administration of ovine Colostrinin (CLN), a proline-rich polypeptide isolated from ovine colostrum, can effectively treat Alzheimer's disease patients. This study aims to determine whether CLN has effects on the aggregation and toxicity of synthetic beta-amyloid (Abeta), implicated as a causative agent of AD. DESIGN AND MEASUREMENTS: Using cell assays, we examined if pre-treatment of neuronal cells with CLN confers protection. RESULTS: The data from cytotoxicity assays (using MTT and LDH) demonstrated that pre-treatment of human neuronal SHSY-5Y cells with 5 microg/ml CLN, for 24 hours, confers neuroprotection against Abeta-induced neurotoxicity. Twenty-four hour pre-treatment with 5 microg/ml CLN was also shown to reduce Abeta 1-40-induced apoptosis in human neuronal cells as determined via qualitative and quantitative apoptosis assays. CONCLUSION: The neuroprotection conferred with CLN pre-treatment was reduced with the Fas ligand (FasL) binding antibody Nok1, suggesting that the effects of CLN may involve a Fas:soluble FasL interaction. These findings indicate that CLN could possibly play a role in the prevention of AD pathogenesis, though the inhibition of Fas-mediated apoptosis.

[160]*

Janusz M, Zabłocka A. **Colostral proline-rich polypeptides - Immunoregulatory properties and prospects of therapeutic use in Alzheimer's disease.** Curr Alzheimer Res. 2009 Nov 26. [Epub ahead of print]

A proline-rich polypeptide complex (PRP), subsequently called Colostrinin (CLN), was first isolated from ovine colostrum, was shown to possess immunoregulatory properties, including effects on the maturation and differentiation of murine thymocytes and humoral and cellular immune responses, both in vivo and in vitro. PRP seems to restore balance in cellular immune functions and is not species specific. PRP is a complex of peptides of molecular masses ranging from 500 to 3000 Da. The polypeptide contains 25% proline and 40% hydrophobic amino acids. PRP shows a regulatory activity in cytokine (IFN, TNF-alpha, IL-6, IL-10) induction and possesses the ability to inhibit the overproduction of oxygen reactive species and nitric oxide. Besides its immunoregulatory activity, PRP also showed psychotropic properties, improving cognitive activity and behavior of old rats, humans, and chickens. The properties of PRP prompted the authors to propose the complex for the treatment neurodegenerative disorders. Beneficial effects of PRP/Colostrinin were shown for the first time in double-blind placebo-controlled trials and long-term open-label studies. The results were confirmed in multicenter clinical trials. A very important property of PRP/Colostrinin is the prevention of Abeta aggregation and the disruption of already existing aggregates. The same properties were expressed by one of PRP's components, a nonapeptide (NP). Moreover, PRP modulates neurite outgrowth, suppresses uncontrolled activation of cells, reduces 4-HNE-mediated cellular damage, and modulates expression in cellular redox regulation, cell proliferation, and differentiation. Its biological response modifying activity can play an important role in its use in the treatment of Alzheimer's disease.

*Note: Abstracts 158-160 are from studies examining the effects of proline-rich polypeptides, also known as colostrinin, on Alzheimer's disease. While proline-rich polypeptides appear to be synonymous with transfer factors based on descriptions of their size and structure from patent applications and manuscripts, as well as their effects on immune function, this remains to be determined in the strictest sense. As such, only three abstracts from studies utilizing proline-rich polypeptides were included here as examples of work on the subject.

Appendix II

New York Times obituary for
Dr. Henry Sherwood Lawrence
(1916-2004)

𝕿𝖍𝖊 𝕹𝖊𝖜 𝖄𝖔𝖗𝖐 𝕿𝖎𝖒𝖊𝖘
nytimes.com

April 8, 2004

H. Sherwood Lawrence, 87, Immunology Pioneer

By LAWRENCE K. ALTMAN

Dr. H. Sherwood Lawrence, a pioneering immunologist who helped found the branch of biology that explores the function of lymphocytes, a type of white cell in blood and lymph nodes, died on Monday in Manhattan. He was 87.

His death was announced by officials of New York University, where he had taught and conducted research for more than 50 years.

Dr. Lawrence, who was known as Jerry, was also an expert in infectious diseases, and his research generated other advances in immunology. Dr. Lawrence conducted research on the way the body rejects transplanted organs and how various conditions can damage tissue.

Dr. Lawrence was best known for his discovery, in 1949, of a substance known as "transfer factor," a product of T-lymphocytes, which play crucial roles in defending against a wide variety of infectious agents.

He named the product after showing that the type of immune response that lymphocytes could transfer to nonimmune animals could sometimes be transferred to enhance the body's defenses.

Transfer factor is a small molecule, and it has been the center of scientific mystery, in part because Dr. Lawrence and other scientists were unable to identify it precisely. Some scientists suspect that transfer factor represents bits of many molecules.

"Although there was significant controversy surrounding transfer factor, Jerry doggedly pursued the concept of immune reconstitution that has become a very important field of immunology," said Dr. Anthony S. Fauci, the director of the National Institute of Allergy and Infectious Diseases.

Dr. Lawrence predicted many aspects of the functioning of lymphocytes and immune cells, and his work provided clues to the later discovery of immune substances known as cytokines.

Dr. Lawrence also identified a link between the way cells respond immunologically to microbes like the bacterium that causes tuberculosis and the type of immune responses involved in the rejection of transplanted organs, said Dr. Fred T. Valentine, an immunologist who worked with Dr. Lawrence at N.Y.U.

Henry Sherwood Lawrence was born in Astoria, Queens. He graduated from New York University in 1938 and its medical school in 1943.

After a year's internship, Dr. Lawrence served in the Navy in World War II as a medical officer aboard a number of ships. He participated in the Normandy invasion at Omaha Beach and in the invasions of southern France and Okinawa, Japan, and received Bronze Stars in each.

After the war, he completed his training as a specialist in internal medicine at New York University and joined its medical faculty in 1949.

In 1959, he became head of infectious diseases and immunology, a position he held until his retirement in 2000. He was co-director of medical services at Bellevue and New York University Hospitals from 1964 to 2000.

Dr. Lawrence was also director of N.Y.U.'s cancer center from 1974 to 1979, and director of its AIDS research center from 1989 to 1994.

Dr. Lawrence was the founding editor of the journal Cellular Immunology and a member of the National Academy of Sciences.

Dr. Lawrence is survived by his wife, the former Dorothea Wetherbee; a daughter, Dorothea Lawrence Browne of New York City; two sons, Dr. Victor John of Greenwich, Conn., and Geoffrey Douglas of Lawrenceville, N.J.; and four grandchildren.

NOTES

NOTES

NOTES

Made in the USA
Lexington, KY
08 April 2013